Strength Training for

About the Author

Michael Fekete, certified coach, strength and conditioning specialist, personal trainer, and master athlete studied and received his training in physical education and physical therapy in Hungary and Canada. He has published numerous health- and fitness-related articles in various strength training and fitness professional publications, and lectures and teaches personal trainers and fitness staff at the YMCA and Sports Clubs of Canada in Toronto, Canada.

He has presented on numerous subjects at fitness conferences and fitness seminars. His specialty is strength training, and one of the main focuses of his practice is to help seniors and the elderly live a physically active and independent life through regular exercise, good eating habits, and an overall healthy lifestyle. As a master athlete, Michael is a world champion many times over. He has won eleven world titles in quadrathlon, kayaking, and outrigger canoeing. In 2000, at age 53, he won the master category in one of the most gruelling international endurance events ever staged, the Extreme Quadrathlon. This is a nonstop multisport race consisting of a 10 kilometer swim, a 40 kilometer kayak portion, 200 kilometers on a bike and a full marathon. Most recently, in July, 2005, Michael competed and won Gold in the World Masters Games. Michael lives in Toronto where he coaches, trains, teaches, writes, and regularly competes in national and international kayaking races.

Praise for Strength Training for Seniors

"Although a book for the lay public, this book is highly referenced with scientific journals. If your senior clients are looking for a credible book to read to help them build their knowledge on strength training, this book is perfect for them."

— *The National Strength and Conditioning Association Bulletin*

"As a practicing physician who has frequent contact with seniors, I fully realize the importance of maintaining fitness, strength and mobility and balance for a safe and improved quality of life. I found this book enlightening and informative and would highly recommend it as a practical source of information and a motivator for seniors to improve their strength and fitness."

— *Seymour Berlin, M.D., CCFP, Toronto, Ontario*

"[The author's] approach to strength training is one of overall well being where health and fitness as well as nutrition and lifestyle are at the basis of a successful training regimen. Strength is a matter of approaching training in the right way and we are sure that [this] book will inspire you."

— *Kayaksport.com*

• • • • • DEDICATION • • • • •

For my mother

Ordering

Trade bookstores in the U.S. and Canada please contact:

Publishers Group West
1700 Fourth Street, Berkeley CA 94710
Phone: (800) 788-3123   Fax: (800) 351-5073

Hunter House books are available at bulk discounts for textbook course adoptions; to qualifying community, health-care, and government organizations; and for special promotions and fund-raising. For details please contact:

Special Sales Department
Hunter House Inc., PO Box 2914, Alameda CA 94501-0914
Phone: (510) 865-5282   Fax: (510) 865-4295
E-mail: ordering@hunterhouse.com

Individuals can order our books from most bookstores, by calling **(800) 266-5592**, or from our website at **www.hunterhouse.com**

Strength Training for Seniors

How to Rewind Your Biological Clock

· ·

Michael Fekete, CSCS, ACE

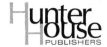

Hunter House PUBLISHERS

> Hunter House Inc., Publishers
> PO Box 2914
> Alameda CA 94501-0914

Library of Congress Cataloging-in-Publication Data
Fekete, Michael.
     Strength training for seniors : how to rewind your biological clock / Michael Fekete. — 1st U.S. ed.
               p. cm.
     Includes bibliographical references and index.
     ISBN-13: 978-0-89793-478-7 (pbk.)
     ISBN-10: 0-89793-478-4 (pbk.)
     1. Physical fitness for older people. 2. Older people—Health and hygiene. 3. Weight training. I. Title.
RA777.6F43 2006
613.7'10846—dc22   2006011152

Project Credits
Cover Design: Jinni Fontana
Book Production: Stefanie Gold
Exercise Photographer: Jonathan Nemethy
Copy Editor: Kelley Blewster
Proofreader: John David Marion
Indexer: Nancy D. Peterson
Acquisitions Editor: Jeanne Brondino
Editor: Alexandra Mummery
Publicist: Jillian Steinberger
Customer Service Manager: Christina Sverdrup
Order Fulfillment: Washul Lakdhon
Administrator: Theresa Nelson
Computer Support: Peter Eichelberger
Publisher: Kiran S. Rana

Manufactured in the United States of America

9 8 7 6 5 4 3 2   First U.S. Edition   12 13 14 15 16

Contents

Important Note

The material in this book is intended to provide a review of information regarding strength training for seniors. Every effort has been made to provide accurate and dependable information, and the contents of the book have been compiled through professional research and in consultation with medical professionals. However, always consult your doctor or physical therapy practitioner before undertaking a new exercise regimen or performing any of the exercises or suggestions contained in this book.

The author, publisher, and editors, as well as the professionals quoted in the book, cannot be held responsible for any error, omission, or dated material in the book. The author and publisher are not liable for any damage or injury or other adverse outcome of applying the information in this book in an exercise program carried out independently or under the care of a licensed trainer or practitioner. If you have questions concerning the application of the information provided in this book, consult a qualified and trained professional.

List of Exercises

Basic Stretches

Acknowledgments

In my studies and everyday aspirations as a trainer, I was guided and influenced by the work of Canadian scholars Roy Shephard and Kenneth Sidney, two of the world's best exercise scientists. Their books, studies, and articles both provided me with insight into the various aspects of aging and motivated me to apply that knowledge for the practical purpose of enabling seniors to become stronger and fitter.

My thanks go to Dr. Tudor O. Bompa, whose excellent books and courses at York University gave direction and cohesion to my ideas regarding strength training.

The greatest professional inspiration, motivation, and encouragement came from my clients, who were able to put up with my unrelenting demands for commitment, discipline, persistence, and focus, as well as with my often unusual training methods while I myself was learning. Through learning and experience, we all became better at training. I was just as happy to see a client who was sedentary and almost disabled get up from a chair and walk as I was delighted to see another win master championships. To each of them I extend my thanks.

Introduction

According to the U.S. Census Bureau, the elderly population (persons age sixty-five and over) in the United States increased elevenfold between 1900 and 1994, but the nonelderly population increased only threefold.[1] This trend will continue into the twenty-first century. Based on the Census Bureau's projections, approximately one in eight Americans were elderly in 1994, but by the year 2030, this ratio will have increased to approximately one in five.[2]

Combine these statistics with the undisputable science linking regular exercise with better health and improved quality of life, and you will understand why increasing numbers of people choose to stay active well into so-called old age (or even to become *more* active than they were in middle age).

This is a book about using strength training to become stronger and to rewind your biological clock for more energy, vitality, well-being, and enjoyment of life.

As a coach, strength and conditioning specialist, rehab specialist, and personal trainer, I have been successfully training seniors for many years. I enjoy knowing that I am a positive force in the lives of others. To see the weak become strong, the sedentary become active, and the disabled and dysfunctional become capable and able is worth more than all the world titles I've won as a master athlete.

This book combines my knowledge of exercise physiology, strength training, overall fitness, motivational psychology, and healthy lifestyle and applies it to the special needs of seniors. A senior who wants to take up strength training—or any exercise program—has needs that are different from those of a younger person. This book specifically addresses those needs.

The benefits of embarking on any exercise program are lessened if the exerciser fails to observe certain underlying principles. The first part of this book lays the foundation necessary to reap the greatest benefits from undertaking a program of strength training. First of all, why strength training? Chapter 1 answers this question by showing why I advocate strength training as among the most beneficial forms of exercise, especially for seniors. Other topics addressed in the early chapters include the physiology of the muscular system, the necessity of obtaining health and fitness assessments before starting an exercise program, some basic healthy lifestyle habits, and the importance of setting goals.

1. F.B. Hobbs, "The Elderly Population," website of the U.S. Census Bureau, www.census.gov/ population/www/pop-profile/elderpop.html (accessed March 12, 2006).
2. Ibid.

The next chapters deal with the specifics of strength training by covering such topics as principles of strength training, elements to include in every exercise session, and how to design your own exercise program. Chapters 9 and 10 contain step-by-step, illustrated instructions for a full compendium of strength-training exercises for the upper body, lower body, and core (abdominal and back area). Since flexibility is an essential component of overall fitness, instructions for basic stretches are also provided. Chapter 11 addresses the differences between training at home and training at a club.

In the final chapters I offer inspiration for seniors by providing real-life stories and my responses to the excuses I often hear for why some people refuse to start an exercise program or why they want to quit one.

Worksheets are provided at the end of certain chapters and again at the end of the book to assist you in applying all of these concepts to your life. They provide structure for taking proactive steps toward modifying your lifestyle, setting short- and long-term goals, and designing your initial strength-training program.

From the very beginning of my career I have been inspired by a statement made by Henry David Thoreau that I read some thirty years ago. It went something like this: "I know of no more encouraging fact than our unquestioned ability to elevate our own life and to promote positive changes in the lives of others by intelligent, persistent, and focused effort, by leaving nothing to chance."

I hope this book not only inspires seniors to train in a safe and effective way to gain more strength, but also provides them with a practical, no-nonsense approach to fitness training in general.

1 | Strength Training
The Way to Rewind Your Biological Clock

> Scientists have yet to discover the philosopher's stone that will confer immortality. However, the ability of regular exercise to reduce biological age by ten to twenty years is no mean miracle. Indeed, I know of no other therapy that could achieve comparable results.
>
> — *Roy J. Shephard*[1]

As one of the many results of social and scientific advancements, we live longer than our predecessors did. Humans' life expectancy has increased dramatically over the last century, and it continues to do so. In 1900 the life span of a male and female living in the United States averaged 48.3 and 51.1 years, respectively. Due to advancements in health care, sanitation, nutrition, and a higher standard of living, by 1990 these figures had increased to 72.1 and 79.0 years, respectively.[2] These are impressive numbers even when we recognize that the full potential for longevity remains far from being realized, due to factors such as pollution, bad eating habits, insufficient exercise, and the increased propensity to acquire certain diseases. But seniors want more than statistical numbers showing a mere extension of life. They want enjoyment, independence, and an enhanced ability to carry on with the activities of daily living, such as caring for themselves. In addition, many of the current generation of seniors actively participate in recreational and athletic activities that they did not engage in before their retirement.[3] They want to live their extra years to the fullest, with vitality and energy.

Whereas a decade ago a senior citizen was expected to slow down and take a rest, now the trend is to add more and more activities to the list of things to do. Wherever you go, you can see seniors on trails, in canoes and kayaks, on bicycles, and in the gym. They are walking, hiking, jogging, playing tennis and golf, taking classes in aerobics, yoga, and Pilates, and engaging in master events in every sport.

Not only do seniors do things they were not supposed to do a few decades ago, but they do them well. A good friend of mine who is eighty years old and several times a master champion in his sport told me a story. He was kayaking on Lake Erie last year, warming up for his training session. He said that as he got older, his bones and muscles needed additional gentle warming up before he was able to paddle hard for a few

1. R.J. Shephard, *Aging, Physical Activity and Health* (Champaign, IL: Human Kinetics, 1997), 29.

2. K.G. Kinsella, "Changes in Life Expectancy 1900–1990," *American Journal of Clinical Nutrition* 55 (1992): 1196S–1202S, www.ajcn.org/cgi/reprint/55/6/1196S (accessed March 9, 2006).

3. R. Krongold, unpublished lecture notes, 2003.

hours on rough water. A group of youngsters paddled by, and he asked if they minded if he cruised with them. They said as a rule they wouldn't mind; however, because they wanted to kayak to an island that was quite a distance away, they would prefer that he didn't. On top of that, they told him they did not like to wait for slowpokes. Les arrived at that island a good thirty minutes ahead of them. He could not hold back a sarcastic remark when he saw them pulling their kayaks onshore: "I had never thought of it before, but now I know how it feels to wait for slowpokes."

Physical activity for seniors is just as important, if not more so, than it is for other age groups. Older adults have come to recognize that the "fountain of youth" is movement. Their desire to exercise is becoming stronger and stronger. Seniors, as an age group, tend to be physically more active than teenagers. The image of sedentary, physically inactive seniors is becoming a thing of the past. Increasingly, senior citizens fully realize that they can't afford to slow down, because they can halt many of the undesirable effects of aging by being physically active. Not only can they check the effects of aging, but they can reverse them. In other words, they can lower their biological age.

What do I mean by "biological age"? Your biological age may be different from your chronological age, which is how long you've actually lived. Based on things like lifestyle, genetics, and medical history, your biological age may be several years younger or older than your chronological age. Although you cannot change your genetics or your past history, you can change your lifestyle, and doing so can have a positive impact on your biological age from this moment forward. As the website RealAge.com puts it, "Science is increasingly showing that certain health choices can slow and perhaps even reverse the rate of aging. Even choices made late in life make a difference. For example, people who exercise early in life, but quit, may show no longevity benefit. In contrast, people who start exercising in their 50s and 60s, or even later, show considerable benefit."[4] This is great news for seniors who are considering embarking on an exercise program.

Recently, Canada took a leading role in recognizing the significance of strength training for older adults when the Canadian Centre for Activity and Aging, funded by a three-year grant from Health Canada, developed strength training guidelines for older adults and published a National Blueprint Document. Canada is also the moving force behind forming an international coalition to draft a document that recommends international training guidelines for seniors. Accepted by the Sixth World Congress on Aging and Physical Activity, held August 3–7, 2004, in London, Ontario, and endorsed by the World Health Organization, these guidelines for safely and effectively strength training seniors will now be implemented all over the world, elevating the quality of life for millions.

4. Website www.realage.com/ company_info/ra_faqs. aspx?pg=1#1 (accessed March 9, 2006).

There have been many books written on various forms of physical training for seniors. In Canada, we are especially fortunate to have some of the most widely recognized international experts on aging and physical activity. They are doing a terrific job of conducting important research, providing fitness professionals with valuable information, and promoting active lifestyles for older adults. These experts are also influencing our governmental and social agencies to invest more money, time, and effort in a national program of making physical activity an integral part of the lives of seniors.

The Importance of Strength Training for Seniors

With all this momentum for a more active adult lifestyle, why is there a need for a book on strength training? Why is strength such an important aspect of our overall fitness?

Strength is the ability to defeat gravity and resistance and to move with vitality and vigor. Strength is the energy that enables us to produce force and to perform skilled and powerful motions. Strength is what prevents the body from giving way, succumbing, crumbling, and failing during its endeavors. *Strength provides the impulse, dynamics, and momentum behind the ability of the human body to act with force and energy.* Without sufficient strength, we would decline and fail. Without strength, we would be unable to perform any of the activities that make us healthy and fit.

General fitness includes strength, endurance, flexibility, coordination, and balance. *However, strength is the basic quality that provides the necessary foundation for and influences our performance of all the other capacities that make up fitness.* Stated more simply, strength affects all other aspects of fitness. It has been established that half of the age-related decline in aerobic capacity is due to a loss of muscle mass.[5] Fortunately, strength can be improved safely and effectively in people of almost any age. It has been demonstrated that even ninety-year-olds can participate in and benefit from serious strength training.[6] Several studies prove that muscle strength can be improved by as much as 66 percent even at a very late age.[7]

General fitness and its most important aspect, strength, decline as we age. One of the effects of this decline is the loss of lean muscle tissue, which means loss of strength. But, through exercise, this deterioration can be slowed down, stopped, and in many cases turned around. All of the effects of enhanced strength through exercise will improve the quality of our lives. Strength is the spring that makes our biological clock tick,

5. S.L. Charette, L. McEvoy, G. Pyka, C. Snow-Harter, and G. Riffat, "Muscle Hypertrophy Response to Resistance Training in Older Women," *Journal of Applied Physiology* 70 (1991): 1912–16.

6. E.N. Booth, S.H. Needen, and B.S. Tseng, "Effect of Aging on Human Skeletal Muscle and Motor Function," *Medicine and Science in Sports and Exercise* 26 (1994): 556–60.

7. T.L. Dupler and C. Cortes, "Effects of Whole Body Resistive Training in the Elderly," *Gerontology* 39 (1993): 314–19.

and, fortunately, this spring can be rewound until a very late age, allowing our clock to tick on vigorously. The seniors I train for strength, and the master athletes I know, not only slow down the process of muscle loss, but also many of them stop and reverse it. But the benefits of exercise are more extensive than this. It is a proven fact that, as opposed to those who do not exercise regularly, physically active seniors enjoy the following benefits of exercise:

1. Better health, including:
   - improved cardiovascular function
   - improved pulmonary function
   - favorable changes in blood lipids
   - improved hormonal activities
   - improved enzymatic activities
   - healthier glucose levels
   - improved immune function and resistance to diseases such as cancer
   - better sleep
   - improved cognitive function
   - increased ability to cope with stress, reduced anxiety and depression, enhanced moods, and an improved ability to relax
   - a more effective immune system
   - social benefits such as increased contacts, friendships, support groups, and involvement in sports events that in turn have positive effects on mental health

2. Better fitness, including:
   - increased strength
   - increased aerobic endurance
   - greater flexibility and range of motion
   - improved coordinative and balancing skills
   - greater velocity of movements (increased muscle speed)
   - healthier body composition (higher ratio of lean muscle to fat)
   - better posture and gait

I could go on at length about the many benefits that elevate the quality of life of active adults. I could also talk endlessly about the various physical and mental/emotional improvements that exercise, in general, has made in the lives of my "mature" clients. But this book is about improving one's strength through serious strength training, so I will deal with the specific benefits of this very important training modality.

Over the years, as a personal trainer and a specialist in strength and conditioning, I have had the opportunity to see and experience the benefits of various exercise modalities, including aerobic training, flexibility training, and strength training. Although I wholeheartedly agree that it is important to balance aerobic, flexibility, and strength training according to the individual needs of each person, strength training is of paramount and primary importance for seniors because, as mentioned earlier, strength has such an important effect on the other aspects of fitness.

I actively train for endurance events that involve swimming, kayaking, biking, and running. At age fifty-three, I won the masters category in one of the most grueling multisport events, the Extreme Quadrathlon, held in Courpière, France. The race involved a 10k swim, 40k kayak race, 200k bike ride, and 42k run—all performed without breaks between events. One would think that for these types of endurance events 90 percent of my training should have been aerobic. However, in fact, it was strength training that was the most important aspect of my exercise regimen. I gained more benefits from strength training than from all other forms of exercise combined. It is a well-known fact in exercise physiology that cardiovascular capacity (expressed in a measurement called VO_2 max) is genetically determined. That means the window for increasing cardiovascular capacity is limited. By contrast, muscle strength and muscle endurance can be dramatically improved through exercise. In fact, with proper training, fast-twitch muscle cells (the kind needed for short bursts of energy) can be converted to slow-twitch muscle cells (the kind needed for strength endurance). I did a lot of cardio training (running, biking, and swimming), and except for improvement in technique, I did not see any improvement in my aerobic capacity. Then I started training the muscles needed for running, biking, and swimming, with a regimen involving a high number of repetitions, a high number of sets, and medium resistance. I saw dramatic improvements in my racing times. It has been established that even marathon runners see dramatic improvements in their racing times after a suitable regimen of strength training.

During the course of my professional career as a coach and trainer, I have used every form of physical exercise to improve the fitness of my clients and of the athletes I train. I have found that strength training brings about the widest range of immediate, maintainable, and long-lasting physical and mental/emotional benefits. Recent research proves that even with the very elderly and the very weak, effective strength training increases independent function skills and produces significant improvements in stair climbing, getting up from the floor, rising from the chair, and walking speed.[8]

What are the physical benefits of strength training in particular?

- Stronger muscles, bones, tendons, and ligaments
- Reduction in the negative effects of osteoporosis
- Improved function, coordination, motor skill, and balance
- Improved range of motion

8. J. Bean, S. Herman, D.K. Kieley, D. Callahan, K. Mizer, W.R. Frontera, and R.A. Fielding, "Weighted Stair Climbing in Mobility-Limited Older People: A Pilot Study," *Journal of American Geriatrics Society* 50 (2002): 663–70.

- Better posture
- Reduction in low-back problems
- Improved body composition, due to an increase in lean muscle mass
- Higher metabolic rate (muscle is the most metabolically active tissue; it burns fat by its mere existence)
- Improved protein synthesis
- Improved cardiac function
- Improved respiratory function, due to an increase in the strength of the chest muscles
- Easing of the pain of osteoarthritis and rheumatoid arthritis
- Better glucose utilization
- Faster gastrointestinal transit
- Decrease in blood pressure
- Improvement in blood lipids
- Improved hormonal and local enzymatic activity
- More effective immune system
- Improved physical appearance

If we compare the physical benefits of strength training to those of exercise in general, we cannot fail to notice that strength training alone affords almost every physical benefit of all other forms of exercise.

Getting Started

Of course, we are able to reap and enjoy the benefits of improved strength only if we practice strength training safely, effectively, and systematically. Otherwise the gains are short-lived and we also run the risk of injuries, burnouts, lack of progress, and, ultimately, failure.

Followed correctly, the program described in this book ensures that all of these fundamentals are met. There is a reason why the exercise descriptions are located *after* the chapters on lifestyle and safety, and *after* the chapters spelling out how to design your initial program based on your health status. *Please do not skip these vital first steps.* Read the book, complete the worksheets, and visit your doctor and a fitness professional to have your health and fitness assessed. Use light weights at first, and take care to start with the beginning exercises (Chapter 9) if you haven't exercised regularly in a while. It is better to start slow and make progress quickly than to start too ambitiously, injure yourself, and be forced to stop training for several weeks.

When beginning a strength-training program, you do not need fancy, expensive, or complicated equipment that takes up too much room, is difficult to move, and is very hard to get rid of. As you will see in the chapters describing various exercises, little equipment is needed for executing an effective strength-training program. Purchase only the basic equipment you need. If, after comparing prices, terms, and the cost of setup at several fitness stores, you buy a flat bench, a set of dumbbells, an exercise mat, and an exercise ball, you will have everything you need to start your strength-training program.

Although machines may be a safe bet for a beginner, especially in a club environment where various distractions can lessen your attention and focus, free weights can be just as safe if you exercise carefully and effectively. Chapter 11 discusses the pros and cons of training at home versus joining a gym. If you decide to train at home, buy a flat bench and a starter set of dumbbells (hand-held weights) weighing three pounds, five pounds, and eight pounds. Men may also want to purchase additional ten- and twelve-pound dumbbells, and you can always buy heavier weights later as your strength improves.

You'll also need an exercise mat for certain trunk exercises and an exercise (stability) ball for core, balance, and functional training. Many companies make stability balls, and they come in various sizes and price ranges. The personnel at the fitness-supply store will be able to recommend one that is most suitable for you.

Beside equipment, you will also need workout attire (T-shirts, sweatshirts, and sweatpants) that does not obstruct movement and that wicks away sweat. You will need a pair of athletic shoes that fit snugly, do not catch on edges, provide ankle support and balance, and are appropriate for strength training. Cross-training shoes or exercise shoes are better for strength training than running shoes because they provide better support.

• • • • •

By picking up this book you have taken the first step toward creating a stronger, more vital you. The rewards you can reap will be well worth the time and energy you devote to improving your fitness. Now let's take the next step toward that goal: learning about the human muscular system.

2 | The Muscular System
Understanding the Basis of Our Strength

Most seniors embark on a strength-training program without bothering to get acquainted with the source of their strength: the muscular system. Aspiring exercisers who are familiar with the location and purpose of their muscles and who have a basic knowledge of the anatomical, physiological, and biomechanical principles behind the muscles' functioning will be more successful in improving their strength. In addition, it is important to acquire a practical knowledge of the terminology used in strength training in order to understand descriptions of exercises and be able to follow instructions.

Muscles: What Are They Good For?

Every movement we make, and an overwhelming majority of our bodily functions, relies on the muscular system. Muscles work almost unnoticed with every heartbeat, with every breath we take, as we stand motionless, and when we sleep. In fact, during every moment of our lives, muscles are performing work.

Besides the ability to perform work, muscles have another essential capacity: Of all the tissues in our bodies, muscles are the best at responding and adapting to the specific demands imposed upon them, and they are able to maintain this ability longer and better than any other organ or bodily system. As a bonus, they also stimulate organs, bones, tendons, ligaments, and the cardiovascular, metabolic, and immune systems to participate in this positive adaptation. The extreme adaptability of muscles and the stimuli they provide for the rest of the body make strength training the most effective form of exercise for the elderly. For a long time, the aging process seemed to be associated with a steady and radical decrease in a person's strength, power, and function. This process can be altered, however, with regular strength training.[1]

1. H. Akima et al., "Muscle Function in 164 Men and Women Aged 20–84 Years," *Medicine and Science in Sports and Exercise* 33 (2001): 220–26.

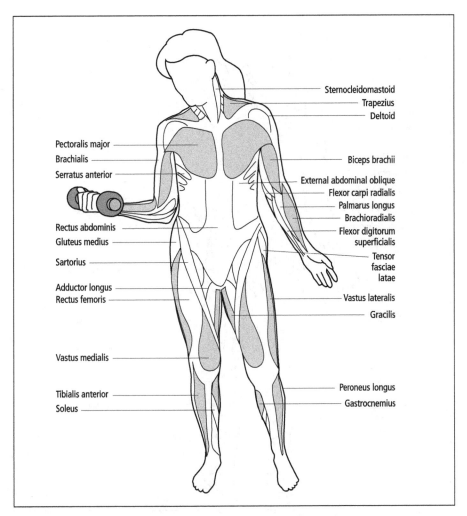

The following labels appear in the figure:

- Sternocleidomastoid
- Trapezius
- Deltoid
- Pectoralis major
- Brachialis
- Serratus anterior
- Biceps brachii
- External abdominal oblique
- Flexor carpi radialis
- Palmarus longus
- Brachioradialis
- Flexor digitorum superficialis
- Rectus abdominis
- Gluteus medius
- Tensor fasciae latae
- Sartorius
- Adductor longus
- Rectus femoris
- Vastus lateralis
- Gracilis
- Vastus medialis
- Tibialis anterior
- Soleus
- Peroneus longus
- Gastrocnemius

FIGURE 2.1. *The musculature of the human body — Front view*

The muscles we are interested in when we talk about strength training are the *skeletal muscles,* which are attached to bones, which serve as levers. Skeletal muscles are the muscles of the arms, the face and neck, the torso, and the legs—generally speaking, the muscles that we use to produce motion and locomotion, and to maintain certain positions (see Figures 2.1, 2.2, and 2.3). Skeletal muscles produce movement of body parts in relation to one another and/or against an outside force or resistance. They create the tension necessary to keep us upright against gravity, to allow us to hold objects, and to maintain correct posture.

Besides skeletal muscle, our bodies contain other muscles that are not attached to bones, for example, the muscles of the heart, called *cardiac muscle,* and the muscles in the walls of organs such as the intestines and stomach, called *smooth muscle.* The primary purpose of these muscles is to help perform specific bodily functions.

Skeletal muscles have an amazing ability to relax, contract, and produce force that results in movement. They respond to exercise, or the lack

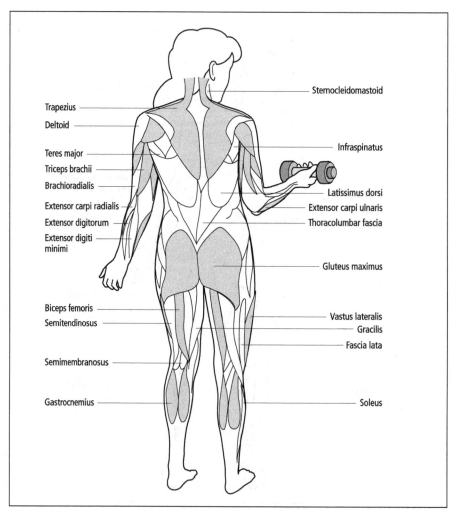

FIGURE 2.2. *The musculature of the human body — Rear view*

of exercise, faster and more efficiently than any other body part or system. Exercise that provides positive stimulus for the muscles will result in bigger and stronger muscles. Lack of exercise will lead to reduced and weaker muscles, and inappropriate exercise will cause injuries, increased wear and tear, and a gradual degradation of the muscular system.

Muscles are attached to our bones via cables that are called *tendons.* Tendons, which are made of a less active form of tissue, transfer energy between the force-producing muscle "engines" and the levers that are our bones. The motion produced usually happens around a joint (or around several joints in the case of complicated movements). Joints, usually located at the ends of the bones, are held together by *ligaments* and are lined and padded with *cartilage,* which acts as a lubricated shock absorber (see Figure 2.4). Because muscle action exerts force on tendons, bones, and joints, muscle work results in positive adaptations not only in the muscles themselves but also in these other tissues. This means that strength training yields both stronger and bigger muscles and stronger

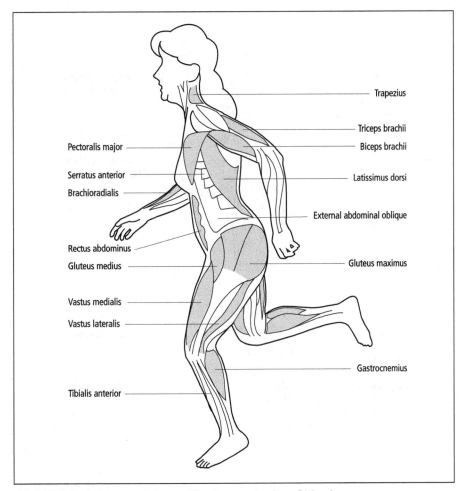

Trapezius

Triceps brachii

Biceps brachii

Pectoralis major

Serratus anterior

Brachioradialis

Latissimus dorsi

External abdominal oblique

Rectus abdominus

Gluteus medius

Gluteus maximus

Vastus medialis

Vastus lateralis

Gastrocnemius

Tibialis anterior

FIGURE 2.3. *The musculature of the human body — Side view*

and more robust bones, tendons, and ligaments. The overall outcome is a greater capacity to perform work as well as an increased protection against injury.

The fuel our muscles use is stored in different forms in the muscles themselves, around organs, under the skin, in the blood, and in the liver. In whatever form and at whatever location this fuel is stored, it has to be broken down through various processes into *adenosine triphosphate* (ATP), which provides the direct energy for muscle action. Just as an engine produces exhaust fumes, our muscles produce various waste products that must be absorbed, processed, removed, and sometimes reused. These tasks are accomplished through a series of different metabolic processes.

Muscle tissue—unlike fatty tissue, bones, tendons, ligaments, and the skin—is a *metabolically active tissue*. In simple terms, this means it burns fuel, even when it is at rest. The amount of fuel used for muscle action is measured in *calories*. While we sleep, our skeletal muscles burn more than 25 percent of the calories we are using. The bigger and more active our muscles, the more calories they burn.

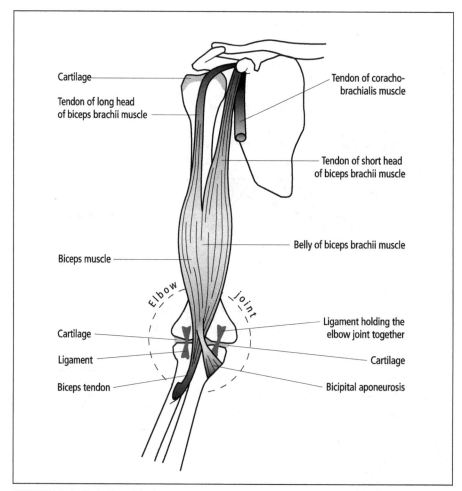

FIGURE 2.4. *Relationship between muscles, tendons, bones, and ligaments in the upper arm*

Muscles are made of *fibers*. The number of fibers in a muscle is genetically determined. An increase in the size of our muscles is the result of extra proteins being built into the individual fibers, rather than the result of an increase in the number of fibers. There are two primary muscle fibers: *slow-twitch* (Type I) and *fast-twitch* (Type II). When we perform cyclical-repetitive movements at a relatively low level of force for a long time—such as distance running, walking, or distance biking (forms of exercise called *aerobic)*—we rely mostly on slow-twitch muscles to do the work. When we produce a high level of force for a shorter period—such as jumping, sprinting, or lifting a heavy weight (forms of exercise called *anaerobic)*—we rely mainly on fast-twitch muscles. During regular strength training, which consists of several *repetitions* performed in several *sets,* both muscle types participate equally in performing the movements.

A large pool of muscle fibers activated by the same motor nerve is called a *motor unit.* When a *nerve impulse* originating from the brain activates a motor unit, all fibers in that unit contract with maximal force. The overall force of the movement produced is regulated by the number of motor units participating in the movement. Depending on the amount of force required to perform a particular movement against a certain resistance at a certain speed, the central nervous system selectively recruits a smaller or a larger number of motor units within the particular muscle or muscle group responsible for executing the movement.

For fine, coordinative, complicated movements performed at a relatively low level of force (such as fastening a button), we use a large number of smaller motor units, found in the arms and the hands. For crude and relatively simple movements performed at a relatively high level of force (such as jumping over a puddle), we use a smaller number of large motor units, such as those found in the legs and the trunk. The major muscles participating in and providing most of the force needed for executing a certain movement or series of movements are called *prime movers*. Those providing assistance through stabilizing the posture required for the movement or helping direct the movement are called *secondary movers*.

How Muscles Do What They Do

Muscle actions that produce a force that defeats a resisting force as the muscle fibers shorten are called *concentric*, or *positive*, actions. Concentric

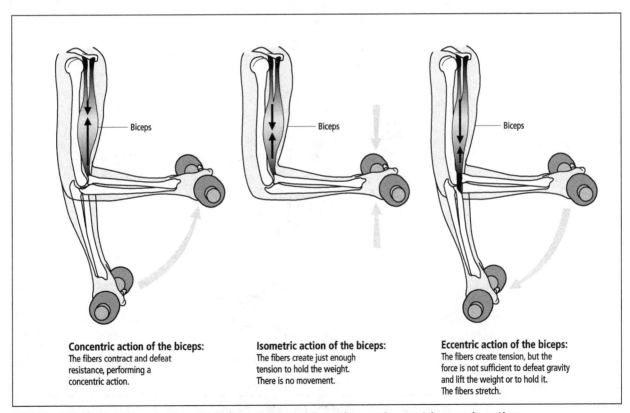

Concentric action of the biceps:
The fibers contract and defeat resistance, performing a concentric action.

Isometric action of the biceps:
The fibers create just enough tension to hold the weight. There is no movement.

Eccentric action of the biceps:
The fibers create tension, but the force is not sufficient to defeat gravity and lift the weight or to hold it. The fibers stretch.

FIGURE 2.5. *Concentric muscle action, isometric muscle action, and eccentric muscle action*

actions involve pushing, pulling, or lifting motions in which body parts move in relation to one another and successfully overcome resistance (see Figure 2.5 on the previous page). Resistance is provided by gravity, and it can be increased by the addition of weights or elastic bands.

Muscle actions that produce a force equal to the resistive force or to the force of gravity but that produce no movement are called *isometric* actions. Isometric exercises include all "holding" actions in which body parts do not move in relation to one another and in which the muscle participating in the action neither shortens nor lengthens but rather maintains a certain tension.

Muscle actions in which the force produced is weaker than the resistive force or gravity and the activated muscle is forced to lengthen are called *eccentric,* or *negative,* actions.

Five fundamental movements result from the contraction (shortening) of muscles: flexion, extension, abduction, adduction, and rotation. There are many other motions and combinations of motions, but to understand

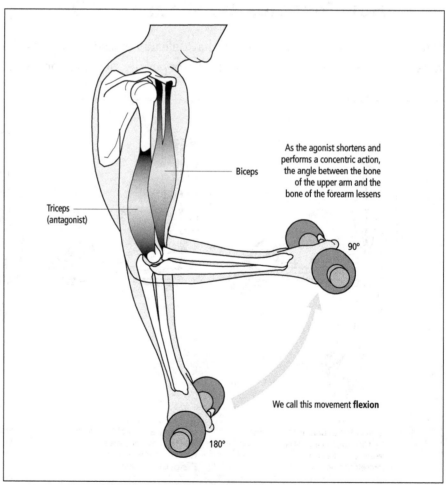

FIGURE 2.6. *Flexion of the arm via the contraction of the biceps muscle (agonist), with the triceps as the potential antagonist*

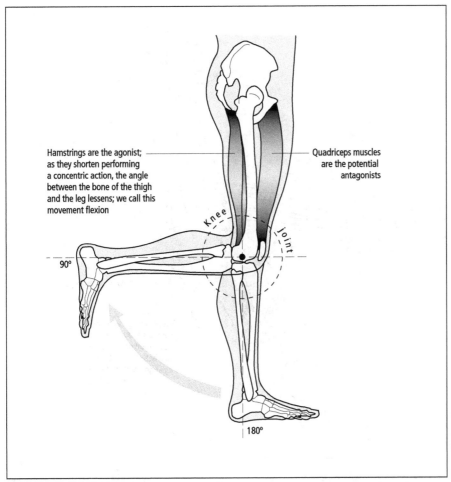

Hamstrings are the agonist; as they shorten performing a concentric action, the angle between the bone of the thigh and the leg lessens; we call this movement flexion

Quadriceps muscles are the potential antagonists

Knee joint

90°

180°

FIGURE 2.7. *Flexion of the leg via the contraction of the hamstrings (agonist), with the quadriceps as the potential antagonist*

the biomechanics of movement, it will suffice to get acquainted with these five basic ones.

Flexion and extension are best observed if we view the person performing the movement from the side. *Flexion* involves decreasing the angle between two bones connected to the same joint (see Figures 2.6 and 2.7). Let us consider the biceps curl. At rest or at the beginning of the biceps curl, the upper arm and the forearm, connected at the elbow joint, are at a 180-degree angle to each other. As we activate the biceps muscles—the muscle performing the desired movement, or *agonist*—the shortening of muscle fibers in the biceps will move the bones of the forearm closer to the bone in the upper arm. In this case, the triceps is the *antagonist* muscle, for it has the potential of opposing the action of the biceps.

Extension involves increasing the angle between two bones connected to the same joint (see Figures 2.8 and 2.9). When we do a chest press, a military press, or a push-up, we increase the angle between the bones of the upper arm and those of the forearm by contracting the triceps

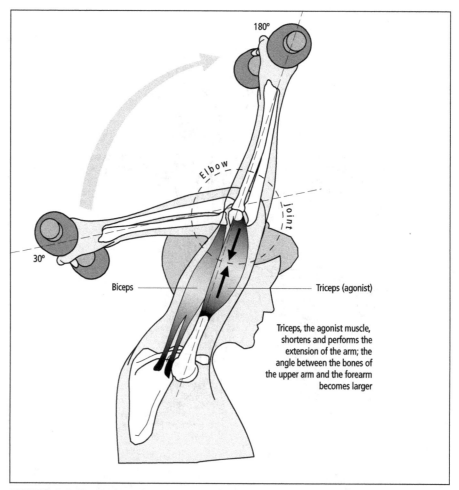

180°

Elbow

joint

30°

Biceps

Triceps (agonist)

Triceps, the agonist muscle, shortens and performs the extension of the arm; the angle between the bones of the upper arm and the forearm becomes larger

FIGURE 2.8. *Extension of the arm via the contraction of the triceps muscle (agonist), with the biceps as the potential antagonist*

muscles. During the execution of any exercises resulting in the extension of the arm, the triceps muscle plays the role of the agonist and the biceps the antagonist.

Abduction and adduction are best observed by looking at the person performing the movement from the front (see Figures 2.10 and 2.11). *Abduction* is a movement away from the midline of the body. When we activate the gluteus medius and gluteus minimus muscles, located on the outside region of the hip, they contract as agonists, and the result is the abduction of the thigh. In common language, we lift our leg sideways, away from the midline of the body.

Adduction is a movement toward the midline of the body. Imagine sitting on a chair with a large exercise ball between your knees. As you squeeze your knees together, you activate the adductor muscles, located in the inner thigh, and they contract, causing both knees to move toward the center. When performing this movement, the adductor muscles (in the inner thigh) play the role of agonist and the abductor muscles (on the outside region of the hip) play the role of antagonist.

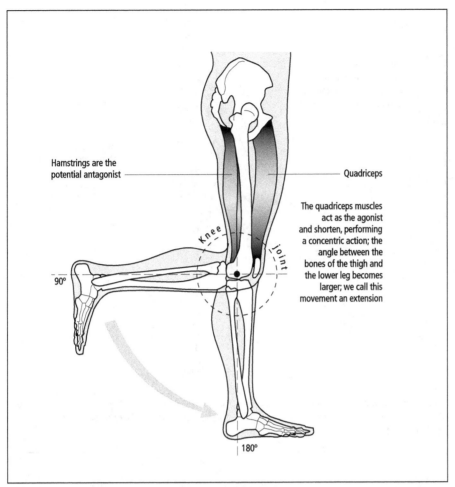

FIGURE 2.9. *Extension of the leg via the contraction of the quadriceps (agonist), with the hamstrings as the potential antagonist*

Rotation is the motion of a bone around a central axis. The most frequently rotated bones are the femur, at the hip joint, and the humerus, at the shoulder. Rotating the trunk around the central axis of the spine is also a form of rotation (see Figure 2.12).

Muscles not only perform movements; they also play an important part in providing natural and neutral alignment of body parts, resulting in healthy posture. Many injuries, both acute and chronic (such as lower-back pain), are caused by an inability to maintain natural alignment and correct posture due to muscle imbalance.

Exercise Terminology

This section lists a few more terms you will encounter as you continue reading this book or when you talk with a personal trainer.

We usually perform any one particular exercise several times to safely and properly stimulate certain muscle groups. Each time we perform a

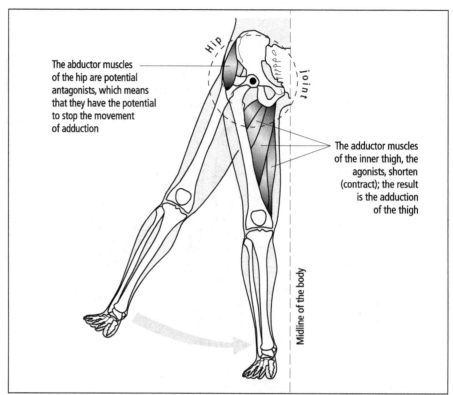

The abductor muscles of the hip are potential antagonists, which means that they have the potential to stop the movement of adduction

Hip
joint

The adductor muscles of the inner thigh, the agonists, shorten (contract); the result is the adduction of the thigh

Midline of the body

FIGURE 2.10. *Adduction of the leg via the contraction of the adductor muscles (agonist), with the gluteus medius and gluteus minimus muscles as potential antagonists*

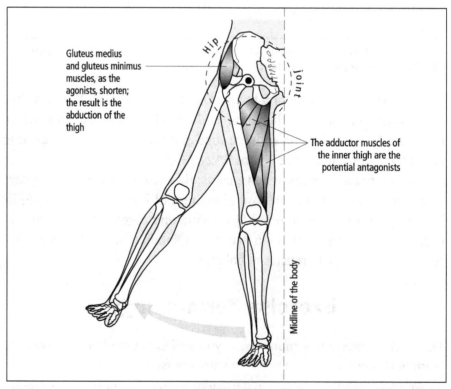

Gluteus medius and gluteus minimus muscles, as the agonists, shorten; the result is the abduction of the thigh

Hip
joint

The adductor muscles of the inner thigh are the potential antagonists

Midline of the body

FIGURE 2.11. *Abduction of the leg via the contraction of the gluteus medius and gluteus minimus muscles (agonists), with the adductors as potential antagonists*

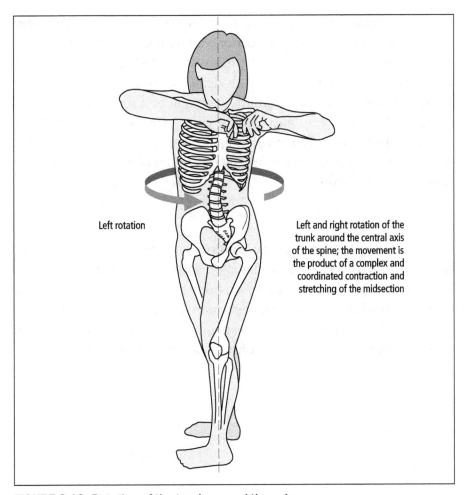

Left rotation

Left and right rotation of the trunk around the central axis of the spine; the movement is the product of a complex and coordinated contraction and stretching of the midsection

FIGURE 2.12. *Rotation of the trunk around the spine*

single prescribed movement—whether it is flexion, extension, rotation, adduction, abduction, or a combination of more than one of these—we are doing one *repetition,* or *rep*. When we perform more than one repetition of the same movement or series of movements, we are doing a *set* of repetitions. If, for example, we perform the prescribed movement eight times in a single set, we are doing a set of eight repetitions. If we perform multiple sets, we might do three sets of eight repetitions.

Muscle fatigue is a temporary phenomenon caused by the depletion of nutrients, lack of sufficient nerve impulse, and an accumulation of lactic acid. It usually occurs at the end of a set of several repetitions. Muscle fatigue and the accompanying discomfort (burn) usually disappear after a short rest (i.e., about a minute). *Muscle soreness,* on the other hand, is a longer-lasting discomfort caused by microscopic lesions or tears in the muscle. Depending on the extent of microscopic damage, forty-eight to ninety-six hours of rest is needed for the processes of repair and rebuilding to be completed. It is these processes that lead to stronger muscles.

Muscle strength is the capacity of a muscle to perform a movement against resistance. Maximum strength is the capacity to perform one movement against maximum resistance. Maximum strength is measured by what is called *one repetition maximum.* I do not recommend that seniors ever test their maximum strength. We are in the business of safely improving our strength, not dangerously demonstrating it. *Muscle endurance* is the capacity to perform a certain movement or a series of movements against submaximal resistance several times, usually up to the point of muscle failure. I also do not recommend that seniors test the limits of their muscle endurance by performing repetitions of an exercise up to the point of muscle failure.

• • • • •

This chapter has acquainted you with some of the characteristics, functions, and biomechanics of the human musculature and has given you a basic knowledge of the terminology used in strength training. In the next chapter you will read about the importance of assessing your health and fitness levels. Without such an assessment, attempting to build stronger muscles would be like trying to construct a building without an architectural plan.

3 | Health and Fitness Assessments

Before you embark on a strength-training program (or any exercise program), it is very important to undergo a health screening by your family doctor and a fitness assessment by a qualified fitness professional. Most would-be exercisers regard these screenings as unnecessary, tedious, and a waste of time. They cannot be more wrong. The care and attention invested in a thoughtful and sensible gathering of all information relevant to your health and fitness will be rewarded by the benefits of a safe and successful exercise program.

Assessing your health and fitness levels reveals your potential and your limitations, both of which are integral parts of getting acquainted with your body. Equipped with the relevant information regarding your health and fitness levels, you will be able to avoid injuries, adverse reactions, and serious complications. By contrast, ignoring this very important aspect of preparation for a physically active lifestyle increases the risk of serious injury, may aggravate existing medical conditions, and may create unwanted new ones.

Besides gathering pertinent information about your medical and fitness status, the goal of these assessments is to identify conditions and medications that may place you at risk when performing certain activities. For seniors in particular, especially those who have been sedentary for many years, these include age-associated conditions such as reduction in muscle and bone mass, declining flexibility and range of motion, the risk of coronary heart disease, high blood pressure, slow reaction time, loss of balance, and the gradual degradation of many other bodily functions. All of these are greatly aggravated by inactivity. Without the information gained from appropriate health and fitness screenings, designing a suitable strength-training program, setting fitness goals, and planning the pace of progress can be risky and ineffective.

The Health Screening

Your family doctor, who is familiar with your medical history and the rate of your biological aging, will be able to advise you of the various risks of a strength-training program and of any possible contraindications (precautions) and limitations you should observe. Once you've been exercising for a while, you'll want to check back with your physician so that he or she can assess the impact of exercise on your health and, if necessary, suggest modifications to your program.

As you know, medications can have adverse side effects. Older adults are especially vulnerable both to side effects and also to interactions between drugs, diet, chronic conditions, and exercise. If you are taking prescription medications such as antihypertensive agents, antiangina agents, anticoagulant agents, antiarrhythmic agents, antilipidemic agents, or digitalis glycosides, you should be aware of their side effects in general and as they relate to exercise specifically. In particular, find out how they can influence the body's response to strength training. Side effects may range from headaches to dizziness, drowsiness, dehydration, increased fatigue, bleeding, easy bruising, and shortness of breath. They may affect balance, increase or decrease heart rate, or mask fatigue. Your physician will be able to provide you with relevant information regarding your prescriptions. Use it to help you plan the nature, frequency, and intensity of your strength-training regimen.

What are the most common medical conditions that can affect an exercise program?

- Various forms of cardiovascular disease, including conditions that can predispose one to cardiovascular disease, such as coronary artery disease, high blood pressure, heart arrhythmia, or unhealthy cholesterol levels
- Various diseases of the kidney, liver, bladder, and digestive tract
- Conditions affecting the nervous system
- Pulmonary and respiratory diseases, such as asthma, bronchitis, and emphysema
- Various forms of degenerative spinal disease
- Joint diseases, such as arthritis
- Conditions such as sciatica

Each of these conditions requires special attention and consideration, and each influences the way you or your fitness professional should design and execute your training program.

The Fitness Assessment

After obtaining a medical clearance and all the information relevant to your health status, the next step is to have a fitness assessment done by a qualified fitness professional. There are various ways to obtain a comprehensive fitness test. Your doctor can arrange for one at a medically approved testing center or clinic, or you can go to a fitness club.

The professional in charge of assessing your fitness status will ask you about your medical history, your fitness and exercise history, the medications you are presently taking, and various conditions that may affect your ability to exercise. He or she will engage you in tests to check your physical responses to various forms of exercise (aerobic, strength, and flexibility). He or she will determine your body composition. After completing a final evaluation of all of your medical and fitness data, he or she will be able to recommend an initial exercise program to get you started.

• • • • •

Once you have acquired a basic knowledge of human musculature (Chapter 2) and have a pretty good idea of your health and fitness status, the next step is to assess your lifestyle habits and make the necessary adjustments.

4 | Healthy Lifestyle Habits
Good Nutrition and Stress Management

If you want to become a stronger and better-functioning adult, it is important to assess your lifestyle habits. The positive return for the time and effort invested in improving your strength and fitness will be multiplied many times if you adopt lifestyle habits that are conducive to health and fitness. *The two most important healthy lifestyle habits are good nutrition and the ability to cope with stress, including the ability to relax.* Take a critical look at your lifestyle habits, assess them, and, where necessary, make suitable adjustments. Otherwise, strength training might add another imposition to an already overtaxed system.

Various methods exist for achieving positive change. Self-declared gurus advocate miraculous methods that they claim will dramatically improve everything about you in a few months. That is something I cannot and will not promise. Rather, I advocate the method that Aristotle recommended when he talked about arriving at a state of excellence gradually through self-improvement. He did not look at achieving excellence as one grand act, but rather as a series of good, small habits.

In the following pages, we will look at these two important components of overall lifestyle. I will explain how they affect your health and fitness and offer tips for making gradual and consistent changes for the better. At the end of the chapter I've included three worksheets: the Behavior-Change Commitment Contract, Stress-Management Strategies, and the Behavioral Balance Sheet. They also appear at the end of the book. I've included them in both locations to increase the chances that you will actually read, contemplate, and complete them. Whether you complete these worksheets now or after you've finished reading the book, you can use them as a hands-on aid for helping you put into practice the ideas set forth in the section on stress management that is located later in this chapter.

A similar aid for putting into practice the advice offered in the next section, which concerns nutrition, is the suggestion I make to keep a food diary while you begin to incorporate healthy new eating habits. Keeping a food diary is a tool you may decide to return to every once in a while, whenever you're ready to make another change for the better.

Nutrition

If you want to build a strong body, you must give it quality materials with which to build. Without proper nutrition, exercise imposes an additional demand on your body.

The dominant form of malnutrition in developed societies is overeating. Both the volume and the caloric content of the food we eat is more than we need for healthy survival. All-you-can-eat buffets, colossal restaurant servings, and jumbo-sized supermarket packaging are evidence of a popular obsession with quantity, and the excess amount of fat that many North Americans carry is the devastating result of this trend. As a result of the combination of overeating, monotonous diet, and lack of activity, by the 1990s obesity had reached epidemic proportions among the elderly. The definition of obesity is far from uniform. In general, a person is considered obese if he or she weighs fifty-five to sixty-six pounds (twenty-five to thirty kilograms) more than the ideal weight for his or her height. Other sources say a person is considered obese who weighs more than 20 percent in excess of his or her recommended weight. Health consequences of obesity range from diabetes to heart disease, from vascular diseases of the brain to flat feet and osteoarthritis of the hips, knees, and lumbar spine. Obesity is associated with high plasma cholesterol, an increased risk of certain cancers, gallbladder disease, and all kinds of psychological problems. For an overweight person, every movement is made at a greater cost, and balance is more difficult to maintain. Obese people cannot move quickly; they lose coordination and risk falls and injuries. Accumulation of fat around the abdomen and underneath the diaphragm restricts circulation and breathing. I could go on endlessly about the adverse effects of being obese.[1]

It is very important that you take a sensible approach to changing your dietary habits, whether your problem is overeating or a poor diet in general. Again, setting realistic goals, achieving gradual improvements, and enjoying the process of achieving them are more conducive to lasting results than dramatic and desperate actions, which usually lead to frustration, disappointment, and, finally, defeat.

Look at what you eat and decide which foods should be eliminated from your diet and which should be introduced into it. Be persistent.

1. R.J. Shephard, *Aging, Physical Activity and Health* (Champaign, IL: Human Kinetics, 1997), 274.

Make a list of dietary goals and work on that list patiently and gradually. Keep a record of what you eat. Be sure to write down every bite you take. Make reasonable decisions based on readily available and proven facts and current nutrition science. *Enjoy the process of becoming a healthy eater instead of suddenly embracing one diet/nutrition fad or the other.* When in doubt, hire a reputable, certified nutritionist. In the next few paragraphs I will outline the basic eating plan I follow. You can use my recommendations as guidelines for a healthy diet.

In the morning I usually eat a bowl of fiber-rich, wholesome cereal. The supermarket shelves contain hundreds of cereals in attractive packaging, some of which have no more nutritional value than the boxes they are sold in. Most cereals contain some form of processed and denaturalized grain, sugar, artificial flavor and color, and other additives. However, also available are a number of healthy and nutritious cereals, rich in fibers and low in sugar and other additives. My favorites are Ancient Grains, Seven Grains, Multigrain, and Fibre First Multi-Bran from President's Choice (a Canadian brand), and All-Bran Buds from Kellogg's, but other manufacturers also produce wholesome cereals. General Mills has recently begun including whole grains in all of its breakfast cereals. I like to add blueberries, papaya, strawberries, or raspberries, and I use either skim milk or soy milk to moisten my cereal.

Another breakfast I like is no-fat, plain yogurt, to which I add papaya, strawberries, blueberries, and/or raspberries. Sometimes I eat eggs scrambled with lots of green pepper, tomato, and onion, and toast made from whole-wheat bread. If I use three eggs, I take the yolk out of two of them. I always drink green tea in the morning.

After breakfast, I prepare my snacks for the day. I put celery stalks, carrots, diced turnips, and sprouts in a sealable bag, and almonds, walnuts, sunflower seeds, and pumpkin seeds in another. I also juice celery, turnips, cucumbers, and beets, put the juice in a bottle, and add some ground flaxseed. I call this strange brew Metabolic Dominance, for I am confident that drinking it helped me win nine world titles in various master events, from kayaking to a quadrathlon. In 1999, at age fifty-two, I won the master category in the Diamond Man Long-Distance Quadrathlon World Championship, in Ibiza, Spain. The event involved a 5k swim, a 20k kayak race, a 100k bike race, and a 21k run (half marathon). After I finished, I was celebrating with my friends when the relay team for the British Royal Marines finished their race. They were all in their twenties, and their team included a swimmer, a kayaker, a biker, and a runner. Performing solo, I had finished the race about two minutes ahead of them. One of them came up to me and asked how it was possible that I had beaten them. "I drink swamp juice," I said and offered him my bottle of juiced celery, beets, carrots, and turnips, which also included ground flaxseed. They tasted it and decided they liked Coke better. The next year I beat them by four minutes. That converted two of them to my Metabolic Dominance.

Throughout the morning I snack on my seeds and greens and drink my swamp juice. For lunch I eat grilled chicken, fish, or turkey, with steamed broccoli, green peas, green beans, and yams, after which I snack until dinner. Early in the evening I have a light dinner, which usually consists of green salad with tofu, olive oil, and lemon juice. I do not snack in the one or two hours before bedtime.

Because I drink plenty of green tea and vegetable juice (my swamp juice) and eat lots of fruit (which is about 90 percent water), I drink only about half a liter of water per day. Counting all the fluids I take in various forms, I probably consume around two liters (half a gallon) of liquid per day. In winter, when the availability of fresh veggies in Canada is limited and when there is less sunshine (which is needed for the production of certain vitamins, such as vitamin D), I take one multivitamin/mineral supplement per day.

If you're wondering whether I ever allow myself a treat, you must understand that my definition of treats differs from the popular one: My ice cream is a cold fruit salad. I occasionally enjoy a piece of organic dark chocolate, I drink an occasional glass of red wine, and once in a while I'll indulge in a plate of spaghetti with meat balls. My idea is that if my overall regimen is dominated by super-healthy food, now and then I can eat spaghetti with meat sauce, or even a slice of pizza. But those are the exceptions. My snacks are also different from the norm: Rather than chips and candy, I regard seeds, nuts, and dried fruits as my snacks.

There are as many eating plans as there are stars in the sky. Even if we discount the fads and unscientific diets, each plan has followers who swear by it. You may prefer one over the other depending on your physiological, psychological, and cultural profile. As long as an eating plan contains foods that are wholesome and natural, and as long as you refrain from eating junk food and from overeating, whatever diet you follow is fine with me.

Besides looking at *what* you eat, you may also want to look at *how* you eat. I always eat relatively little at any one time. I try to eat slowly. I chew my food well—digestion starts in the mouth. If I eat quickly, the message to the brain indicating that I have eaten enough is usually late and, before it registers, I have already overeaten.

There is nothing magical about my diet. My philosophy is quite simple. I like eating good, wholesome foods because I know they are an important factor in my health and fitness, and I prefer health and fitness to illness. I avoid overeating because I like to be lean and slim a lot more than I like being fat. I stay away from the attraction of easily available bad foods because I know that the price I pay for giving in to the temptation of taste and convenience will be high. I do not fall for fads because the bogus science they are based on does not make any sense to me.

Of course, there are some people who, for one reason or another, need a stricter dietary regimen as prescribed by a qualified nutritionist. If this is true for you, you will probably be required to keep a record of what and how much you eat, which is a good idea.

If you cannot afford the services of a registered nutritionist, you may want to look into an eating plan such as the one advocated by Dr. Dean Ornish, or choose a reasonable popular diet such as the South Beach Diet. Books on both are available in your local bookstore. *Stay away from fads and charlatans who promise spectacular and dramatic changes but fail to inform you about the health costs and the impossibility of maintaining the results over the long term.*

Furthermore, do not listen to pseudoscientific humbug recommending the elimination of carbohydrates from your diet. Many foods contain nutritious complex carbohydrates, which slowly and gradually diffuse energy throughout the body. When including carbohydrates in your diet, look for foods with a low *glycemic index*. The glycemic index (GI) is a ranking of carbohydrates according to their immediate effect on glucose (blood sugar) levels. Carbohydrates that break down quickly during digestion have the highest glycemic ratings. The body's response to these carbs is to rapidly increase glucose levels. Carbohydrates that break down slowly, releasing glucose gradually into the bloodstream, have low glycemic ratings. Foods that have a low GI include beans, lentils, chickpeas, barley, legumes, nuts, seeds, and whole-wheat or multigrain bakery products.

With glucose assigned a GI of 100, nutritionists rank foods with a low, medium, or high glycemic index according to the following ranges:

- Low GI = 55 or less
- Medium GI = 55–69
- High GI = 70 or more

A table containing the GIs of some common foods is available at the following website: www.diabetesnet.com/diabetes_food_diet/glycemic _index.php.

Here are some additional points to keep in mind about the glycemic index:

- Eating foods with a low GI will result in a less significant rise in blood glucose levels after meals.
- A low GI diet can help you lose weight.
- Low GI foods can improve the body's sensitivity to insulin.
- A low GI diet can improve diabetes control.

- Low GI foods keep you feeling full longer.
- Low GI foods can prolong physical endurance.

Also, avoid any advice that recommends eliminating all fat from your diet. Certain essential fatty acids, found in deep-sea fish oil, flaxseed oil, and other oils, are absolutely necessary for maintaining a healthy body.

The most effective way to improve your eating habits is to gradually eliminate bad foods and gradually introduce more wholesome foods into your diet. Eliminating unhealthy foods will mean that you need to learn how to read nutritional labels, because some of the items you'll want to avoid are only obvious when you look at the list of a food's ingredients.

Eliminate:
- Hydrogenated or partially hydrogenated oils (trans-fats)
- Soft drinks/sodas
- Sweets and candies
- High-fructose corn syrup

Drastically reduce:
- Saturated fats
- Processed foods
- Red meat
- Full-fat dairy products
- Salt
- Simple carbohydrates that have a high glycemic index, such as dates, fruit rolls, waffles, white bagels and other bakery products, doughnuts, french fries/potatoes, cornflakes, corn syrup, white sugar, honey
- Alcohol

Add:
- Dark-green leafy vegetables, such as spinach, chard, turnip greens, mustard greens
- Cruciferous vegetables, such as bok choy, broccoli, Brussels sprouts, cabbage, cauliflower, collards, kale, kohlrabi, rutabaga, turnips
- Sprouts
- Hummus
- Fresh vegetable juices
- Seeds and nuts
- Legumes, such as lentils, peas, beans
- Fruits, such as berries, papaya, apple, apricot, watermelon, citrus
- Healthy oils, such as the omega-3 oils found in fish oils and flaxseed oil

- Protein-rich, healthy foods, such as tofu and other soy products, fish, turkey, and egg whites
- Skim-milk products, such as fat-free plain yogurt and skim milk

Bad habits, such as smoking, drinking, and consuming products that contain caffeine, also interfere with your goal of getting fitter.

In addition to overeating, another common form of malnutrition in industrialized societies is a monotonous diet. This means that the food many of us eat lacks quality, variety, and balance and is deficient in vitamins, minerals, fiber, and essential fatty acids. It is common knowledge that processed foods are devoid of healthy nutrients and loaded with preservatives, coloring, and taste-enhancing agents that are a source of empty calories and may be harmful to your health. Processed foods lack natural vitamins, minerals, and essential fatty acids—and they may be toxic as well. By "toxic," I do not mean that they contain poisons that will kill you in days. Rather, if they are habitually eaten over a long period, they may lead to chronic bad health. Excess consumption of processed sugar (the most commonly used additive) can eventually cause diabetes, among other illnesses. In particular, sugar in the form of high-fructose corn syrup has been shown to interfere with the body's metabolism, resulting in an even higher risk for type-2 diabetes and other metabolic conditions. Another common additive, salt, can cause high blood pressure in some people. Sugar and salt are present in nearly all processed and canned foods. Most people do not know that just one can of chicken noodle soup (or two pickles) contains the total daily recommended intake of salt. In addition, there are the myriad chemicals added to processed foods to prevent them from drying, aging, turning hard, or changing color.

Another problem with processed foods is that as they are degermed and heat-treated, stabilized and converted, the foods' naturally occurring fibers, enzymes, and important phytochemicals (plant substances that provide nutrients) are removed. In short, most processed foods are denaturalized. They provide easily available empty calories that play havoc with a person's blood sugar, cause bloating, increase body weight, clog the digestive system, and fail to impart the vigor and vitality needed to resist diseases. The number-one step you should take on your way to a healthier life is to slowly but consistently reduce the amount of processed foods you eat. You cannot exclude everything, but you can do a pretty good job of eliminating the worst.

The best way to reduce obesity and improve body composition is to combine exercise and good eating habits. A well-designed program of physical activity accompanied by improvements in your dietary habits will work better than either exercise or diet alone. Attention to good eating habits will provide all the quality-building materials an exerciser needs to build a fit and healthy body, and exercise will ensure that the food is used efficiently rather than being deposited as fat, plaque, excess waste products, and bodily fluids. It has been proven that the many metabolic effects of regular exercise include enhanced protein synthesis, faster gastrointestinal transit time, elevated basal metabolic rate (the number of calories you burn at rest), and better absorption of vitamins and minerals. The overall effect is a loss of fat and a gain in lean, functional muscle mass.

Stress Management

Besides gradually improving my eating habits over several years, I've acquired other good habits and skills that have helped me achieve and maintain a healthy mind and a healthy body. I find that my ability to cope with stress and my capacity to relax are very important parts of my overall strategy for health and fitness.

In your younger years you may have been able to ignore the signals and suppress some of the manifestations of stress and function normally to a certain degree, but generally at approximately age fifty a person begins to pay the price of the cumulative effects of stress. In his famous book, *The Stress of Life,* Hans Selye, who coined the word "stress" and founded the Canadian Institute of Stress, describes stress as a complex chain of internal reactions that occur when we perceive a threat to our existence or well-being. *Excessive stress occurs when the level of aggravation we are experiencing exceeds our capacity to absorb and to deal with the demands imposed upon us.*

Stress had its role in evolution when early human beings had to confront all kinds of physical danger. It was part of the fight-or-flight response: The brain suddenly focused on the threat. Forgetting everything else, the heart began to beat faster, adrenalin was pumped into the blood, arteries dilated, and stored energy supplies were rapidly mobilized as the body went on high alert.

Fear for our physical survival has long since been replaced by fear of losing control. *In developed societies the primary stressors are mental and emotional.* They arise mostly from our interactions with people or from dealing with situations in which we perceive that we have little or no control. They can be challenging and stimulating if we can respond to them healthily and effectively, but they can also be threatening and overwhelming if we perceive them as such. These stressors and the psychological stress they create impact our health and well-being in many ways. *The impact of psychological stress and the resulting negative emotions affect not only our nervous system in the form of nervous agitation, irritation, depression, and anxiety, but they also affect the behavior of almost every cell in our bodies.* Chronic stress destabilizes the body's homeostasis and upsets the body's chemical balances; in short, it disrupts our entire system. As a result, the functioning of the whole body degrades. If the amount, duration, and intensity of stress are more than we can absorb and react to in a healthy manner, the consequences may range from headaches to ulcers, from depression to substance abuse, from the suppression of our immune system to high blood pressure and heart disease. The negative reactions to cumulative stress may manifest themselves in flare-ups of rheumatoid arthritis, in deposits of fat around the abdomen, in disruption of the delicate balance between brain and endocrine system (which makes and releases hormones), and in the release of harmful compounds that cause inflammation. In short, *stress reduces our strength and our ability to maintain a healthy physique.*

The problem is that we can be subject to anxiety, depression, and physical symptoms as a result of prolonged and unabated stress without experiencing any obvious sense of discomfort. For some of us, stress has been such a constant, unremitting fact of daily life that we fail to recognize it as one of the most dangerous and harmful assaults on our well-being. This inability to be aware of what is happening to us may lead us to take on extra stress instead of trying to find a way to cope with it in a healthy and effective manner. At a certain point in everyone's life, *the cumulative effects of stress on body and mind will become so overwhelming that almost any negative experience can trigger an avalanche of adverse reactions.* When this happens we may find ourselves vulnerable to a variety of mental and physical ailments.

We cannot avoid all the stressors in our daily lives. However, we can develop skills to cope with them so that they will not play havoc with our mental, emotional, and physical well-being by creating a fierce civil war between an unbalanced mind and a weak body. *The timely recognition of stress signals and destructive patterns is the most important first step in dealing with stress.* Without first recognizing the manifestation of stress in our lives, we are prevented from taking action against it, and, in a relentless cycle, we remain vulnerable to life's stresses.

Emotional signs of being overwhelmed by stress include the following:

- Irrational fear
- Irritation
- Anger
- Worry
- Nervousness
- Loss of sense of humor
- General negativity
- Emotional exhaustion
- Instability

- Lethargy
- Depression

Behavioral changes resulting from excess stress include the following:

- Pacing and talking to oneself; arguing with imaginary or actual persons who are not present
- Overeating, rushed eating, loss of appetite
- Missed appointments
- Swearing
- Negative self-talk
- Outbursts of anger
- Nagging others
- Sudden increase in bad habits, such as smoking or drinking alcohol or caffeine
- A desire to work more and an increase in the number of mistakes made while working
- Withdrawing, avoiding others, and wanting to be alone

Physical signs of excess stress include the following:

- Tightness in the neck, shoulders, throat, or chest
- Slumped posture
- Headaches
- Strained face
- Shaky hands
- Sweating
- Rapid and shallow breathing
- Dry mouth
- Physical weakness
- Skin rashes

The second step is to identify the causes of stress that elicit adverse reactions and deal with them appropriately. Among the most common sources of stress are personal ambitions, certain perceptions about reality or the nature of things, unreasonable expectations, preoccupations, and over-reaching, which result in a loss of control.

It is not easy to identify sources of stress. Doing so takes self-knowledge as well as the ability to admit that most of the time we humans are not passive sufferers but rather are active promoters of our own stress. This admission requires that a person take action to modify or eliminate certain behavioral patterns that work against his or her well-being. A person may have little faith in his or her ability to do that. He or she may also have to seek advice, which many regard as an admission of weakness. What most people do is they ignore and try to further suppress their symptoms, much like the character in the Woody Allen movie who proudly proclaims that he never shows anger—he grows ulcers instead.

I learned that instead of ignoring and suppressing the symptoms, I should listen carefully to my body and improve my skills for dealing with stress. Stressors do not go away, and symptoms cannot be endlessly suppressed. We must find ways of coping with them. I was past fifty-five when I acquired the proper mindset and tools to cope with life's stresses. Let us talk about the mindset first. Here are my definitions of positive and negative mindset:

Positive mindset is an effective and established system of conscious control of my mental and emotional processes that enhances my well-being.

Negative mindset is the lack of such an established system or the presence of a system that works against my well-being.

I recognized that without conscious control of my thoughts and emotions, I am a wavering creature of moods, easily thrown off judgment and purpose, a specialist in misunderstanding. Without conscious control of my thoughts and emotions, my reactions are reflexive, impulsive, and counterproductive. I get easily preoccupied with useless notions and feelings, and I become resigned to irrational, undesirable, and counterproductive behavioral patterns. Without conscious control of my thoughts and emotions, I enhance my weaknesses instead of reducing them. The end result is defeat and capitulation to life's stresses.

Fortunately, I also recognized that if I persist in patiently adjusting my mindset in the direction of the positive, and if I keep strengthening, conditioning, and honing it, I have a pretty good chance of meeting the challenges presented by life's stresses. From experience, I learned that *a positive mindset is the most powerful conscious force I can employ in regulating the way I use my energy so that it benefits myself and others.*

What are the qualities that make one's mindset positive? They include being able to

- think in a calm, pacified, and reflective manner instead of being disturbed, agitated, and impulsive in one's reactions
- put ideas together rationally and arrive at the right judgment even in the absence of obvious evidence or proof
- decide, plan, and execute a course of action in a patient, persistent, and disciplined manner
- recognize changes and be flexible in adapting to them

- observe and perceive things with a sense of humor instead of outrage, indignation, and anger
- let go of useless and counterproductive thoughts, desires, and ambitions instead of being preoccupied with them
- relax and meditate or rest
- resist temptation and coercion

Do I have a mindset that is characterized by all these qualities? Certainly not, but by trial and error, by falling on my face and getting up again, I constantly improve my mindset.

What are some practical skills for coping with stress in a positive way? Through practice and patience, everyone can develop and enjoy his or her own techniques for dealing with stress. The one I use most frequently is breathing. It is the most readily available and easiest to use tool in my toolbox. As soon as I feel worry, tension, anxiety, anger, or any other negative feeling, I start deep, abdominal breathing. I inhale deeply and hold my breath for a few moments. Then I exhale fully and stretch my diaphragm by expanding my chest without inhaling for another few moments. Then I do another deep, abdominal inhalation (see Figures 4.1 to 4.3 on the next page). I completely focus on this breathing exercise, trying to maximize the volume of air I inhale and trying to exhale fully.

I use breathing regularly to calm my mind and my senses. I do breathing exercises at least six or seven times daily, and I do them before every race. I always deep-breathe when I walk. I find deep breathing both relaxing and energizing. It provides the perfect combination of aerobic exercise and relaxation. It is almost impossible to be anxious while breathing in the manner described above. Besides affording mental relaxation, deep breathing also helps lower blood pressure and improve circulation and digestion.

I have a particular breathing exercise for each stressor. Someone recently asked me how I handle stress, and I answered that I have special breathing exercises for it. When he looked at me incredulously, I jokingly added that I have about twenty different breathing exercises to help me cope with family members, including myself. In fact, out of that twenty, at least ten help me tolerate myself.

The second way I deal with stress is through rest. I have the tendency to run all day and to work on various projects until I drop, accumulating such a deficit of sleep and rest that it seriously affects my well-being. I have to focus on slowing myself down, and the best way to do so is to take a siesta during my working day. I do some breathing exercises, then I lie on the floor with my feet on an exercise ball. I park my thoughts one by one so I can relax both brain and body for about half an hour.

My third tool is using small, sensible solutions to deal with problems and situations that I cannot avoid or tolerate. Here are a few examples:

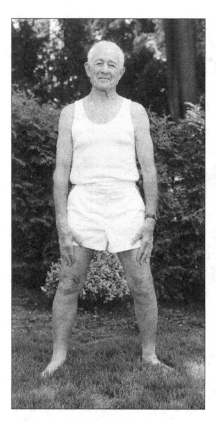

FIGURE 4.1. *Starting position: Stand with your feet shoulder width apart and your arms in a relaxed, extended position. The palms of your hands should gently touch the sides of your thighs.*

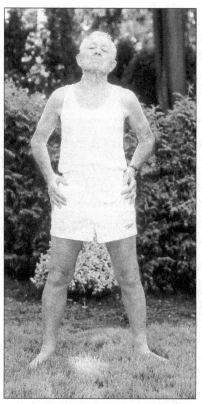

FIGURE 4.2. *Inhale: Begin inhaling slowly, first into the abdomen and then into the chest. At the final stage of the inhalation, expand and lift the chest as much as you can. You can assist the expansion of the rib cage by press-ing your hands against your thighs. Hold the breath for a few moments.*

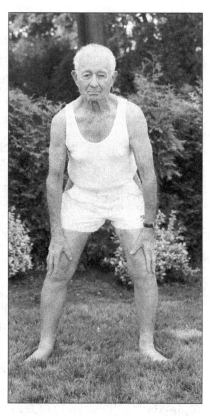

FIGURE 4.3. *Exhale: Begin exhaling by slowly contracting the abdominal muscles and compressing the chest. At the final phase of the exhalation, lean forward and rest your hands above your knees.*

- I do not like to wait, so I always carry a book with me to read.
- I do not like to be stuck in traffic, so I keep a collection of classical music in the car to play when it happens.
- I always carry a notebook because I tend to forget things and then get upset about it.

We all grow older, but it is by no means certain that we will all grow up. Some of us cannot get rid of the childish tendency to believe that life conspires to make us happy or miserable. This immature pattern of thinking, which leads to unnecessary aggravation, can follow us well into old age. It took me some time to grow up and accept the fact that some things just happen. Among the mental processes I use to cope with stress is to adjust my perception to consciously interpret things that are in some way or another directed at me and that appear threatening, insulting, and unreasonable as funny, silly, incidental, and something to laugh at. I view them with a sense of humor. I look for a reason to smile, laugh, or just quietly amuse myself instead of being outraged, indignant, insulted, or threatened.

With conscious control, I can adjust my perception and overcome the compulsion to react at all. I reflect instead. I used to respond immediately to every proposal, question, or provocation with agreement or disagreement. Now I feel free to say that I do not know and that I will have to think about it. I also feel free to ignore whatever I find unreasonable or inappropriate or both.

I never try to be perfect. I always try to do the best I can under the circumstances, but I am not obsessed by the desire to be perfect. Nor do I expect others and the world to be perfect. I look at greater perfection as something I work toward, and I enjoy the process of improving myself, but I never entertain the illusion that I will achieve perfection.

Because this book is about strength training, I do not want to deal more than necessary with the topic of stress management. At the same time, I cannot emphasize enough that *without exercising the mind and training it to cope with stress, one cannot realize half of one's potential to become physically stronger.* Take some time to review the three worksheets that follow. The first one, Behavior-Change Commitment Contract, as the title implies, asks you to make a contract with yourself, specifically about how you will incorporate stress-management techniques into your life. A self-contract is a simple but effective tool for adhering to any plan of action. If you've written down your plan in the form of a contract with yourself, you're more likely to honor it. For the second and third worksheets, Stress-Management Strategies and Behavioral Balance Sheet, you may find that you want to think about them and return to them over the next several days and weeks. You may change or build on your original answers as you get in the habit of self-observation and as you gain more insight into yourself.

• • • • •

At this point, you have acquired a basic knowledge of the human musculature. You have been cleared by your doctor and assessed by a fitness professional. You know that good nutrition and healthy lifestyle habits are just as important as physical training when it comes to your well-being. You've made a contract with yourself to begin incorporating healthy lifestyle habits into your daily routine.

The next step is to set realistic and achievable goals that also challenge and motivate you. In the next chapter, we will deal with the importance of goal setting.

Behavior-Change Commitment Contract

I, _____, will begin my behavior-change program immediately and will incorporate the following into my daily routine:

1. I will pay attention to physical, behavioral, mental, and emotional signs of stress. I will become aware of and record my typical adverse reactions to stress, which may include everything from overeating to negative feelings.

2. I will begin to identify the *sources* of stress in my life and learn to be aware of them as they occur.

3. I will steadily work on improving my personal skills to cope with stress that results in fear, impulsiveness, anxiety, anger, preoccupation, and other negative feelings by

    a. working on building a positive mindset that includes changing perceptions, reactions, and being more reflective rather than reactive
    b. using breathing, relaxing, meditating, reading, listening to music, etc., to prevent and cope with stress
    c. constantly reviewing and appreciating the progress I am making and rewarding myself for making that progress
    d. enlisting the services of a professional counselor if I need outside support to do any of the above

4. I will work for change by taking small, manageable steps, rather than setting myself up for disappointment by trying to make sweeping changes.

_____   _____

SIGNATURE   DATE

Stress-Management Strategies

1. I listen to what my body is telling me. I learn to recognize the following signs of stress:
    - Muscle tightness
    - Slumped posture
    - Shaky hands
    - Sweating and/or night sweating
    - Headaches
    - Dry mouth
    - Rapid and shallow breathing
    - Lack of energy
    - Strained face

2. I am aware of the following behavioral signals of stress and their sources:

Signal	Identify Source
Talking to myself	_____
Arguing with people who aren't present	_____
Overeating/rushed eating	_____
Swearing	_____
Outbursts of anger	_____
Nagging others	_____
Increase in bad habits	_____
Withdrawing	_____
Working more and making mistakes	_____

3. I am aware of the following emotional signs of stress and their sources:

Signal	Identify Source
Fear	_____
Anger	_____
Worry	_____
Loss of sense of humor	_____
Irritation	_____

4. I employ the following strategies to manage my stress:
    a. Change my perception of things; acquire a sense of humor
    b. Reduce ambitions, lower expectations, become more realistic and accepting
    c. Learn to say no
    d. Get adequate sleep and rest
    e. Do deep breathing and use various relaxation techniques
    f. Seek counsel
    g. Others (write them here)

Behavioral Balance Sheet

Under the "Comments" columns, note when you feel each emotion (see the first example)

Positive	Comments	Negative	Comments
1. Sense of humor	e.g., I laugh at myself when I make a mistake.	1. Fear	e.g., I feel fear when I go for a checkup.
1. Sense of humor		1. Fear	
2. Calm		2. Anxiety	
3. Ability to reflect		3. Nervousness	
4. Ability to say no		4. Outrage	
5. Assertiveness		5. Indignation	
6. Optimism		6. Preoccupation	
7. Patience		7. Impatience	
8. Disipline		8. Pessimism	
9. Awareness		9. Annoyance	
10. Ability to let go		10. Worry	

5 | The Importance of Setting Goals

We seem to set mental limits on the possible boundaries of our world and then to work within those limits.[1] We tend to accept certain prescribed beliefs about ourselves and our potential. At the same time, we are also able to imagine ourselves in pursuit of a goal, and we have the capacity to plan how to attain it.

We have a choice. We can either be passive objects of the whims of fate, or we can be proactive in making ourselves what we want to be. When you decide to embark on a healthy and physically active life, you must set realistic and reasonable goals. To achieve those goals, you devise a game plan, a process based on a method.

By nature, we humans are motivated by goals. Mentally and emotionally we want an improved existence; we seem to continually visualize and imagine a greater perfection for ourselves. Our whole conscious life is based on setting our sights on a goal or a set of goals and organizing our activities toward achieving them.

Without goals, our actions would lack concreteness, direction, and focus. Positive attitudes would fade, discipline would erode, commitment would diminish, the temptation to give up would prevail over the motivation to continue, and a fear of failure would win over a determination to succeed. A sensible goal is a realistic target that we consciously aim to reach. Once it has been set, we must remain committed to it. It becomes the purpose behind our activities, strengthening them by adding discipline, intelligence, and consistency. We cannot overestimate the inspirational value to our psyches of setting goals.

Goals for Physical Fitness

If we want to improve our physical fitness, it is very important that we set realistic short-term and long-term goals for ourselves. In doing so, of

1. R.E. Ornstein, *The Psychology of Consciousness* (New York: Penguin Books, 1986), 1.

course, we must take into account the current status of our health and fitness levels. *Our goals must be difficult enough to challenge us, but also realistic enough to be achievable.* We must be convinced that the price of our goals—that is, the time, effort, and care we invest in accomplishing them—is worthwhile and that the goals will eventually lead us to a better quality of life: more fun, enjoyment, and independence.

When it comes to strength training, short- and long-term goals are different for each person. However, all goals that lead to success, in whatever area of life, have several things in common. They are motivational, concrete, and precise. A goal can be as simple as getting up from a chair without assistance or as challenging as becoming a champion master athlete. In some cases, a goal begins as a desire to perform basic functions better and progresses into accomplishing truly exceptional feats. I have had several elderly clients (who now would vehemently resent the description "elderly") whose initial goals were to be able to do daily activities more easily. They surprised themselves by going from being sedentary to becoming master swimmers, kayakers, canoeists, or triathletes.

One of my clients, who started training with me at age fifty-eight, had high blood pressure (for which he was on medication), high cholesterol, and was obese (240 pounds). Within a year, his blood pressure was normal (his doctor took him off medication), his cholesterol was normal, and he had lost fifty pounds. He began to participate in various outdoor recreational activities such as outrigger canoeing, road biking, and hiking. In another year he started adventure racing.

Another client of mine had extreme osteoporosis, bad posture, atrophied muscles, and below-normal strength (she could hardly stand up from a sofa). After two years of progressive strength training she gained lean muscle tissue, her bone mass and bone mineral density substantially improved, and her posture was corrected. She could actively garden, she hiked on weekends, and she joined the local bowling club—all at the age of sixty-six.

I include these stories to help you brainstorm about the possibilities you may wish to envision for yourself. It isn't feasible to give a complete list of personalized goals in a book; however, this section offers guidelines for helping you set some goals for your fitness program. The idea is to start with simple, realistic, and achievable goals and raise the standard gradually and sensibly. What is most important is enjoying the step-by-step process of reaching your goals.

The general, long-term goal of strength training is to become stronger. To progress consistently, you need to commit yourself to a few initial short-term goals that are achievable within two or three months. These short-term goals must be specific, measurable, attainable, relevant, and time-bound. At the end of this chapter, and again at the end of the book, you'll find an Exercise/Lifestyle Commitment Contract. Use it to summarize your goals for the next two or three months (and, later, your goals for a year from now) and to outline a plan for achieving them. This is a very important part of your success strategy. It is also important to reaffirm on a daily basis your belief in your ability to reach these initial goals.

Let us say, for example, that you are about twenty-five pounds overweight. You eat too much red meat, too many processed foods, and too much sugar in the form of sweets. You can perform five parallel squats with your body weight and five biceps curls with a ten-pound dumbbell. You have a problem coping with stress and are easily angered.

In your commitment contract, you pledge to lose ten pounds in three months by reducing your consumption of red meat, processed foods, and sweets and increasing your consumption of fresh green vegetables, fiber-rich foods, and skim-milk products. You pledge to strength train three times a week, for forty-five minutes each time, according to a comprehensive program of lower-body, trunk, and upper-body exercises. Your goal is to perform ten parallel squats with your body weight and twelve biceps curls with a ten-pound dumbbell. Through breathing exercises and other suitable coping and relaxation strategies such as walking, meditating, and resting, you will learn to diffuse and prevent potential angry reactions instead of suppressing them.

These realistic short-term goals will complement each other. Eating wholesome foods that are lower in calories but higher in nutritional value will both help you lose weight and provide better-quality materials for building lean muscle. More lean muscle will increase your basal metabolic rate, which will cause you to burn more calories, even at rest. Losing weight will make it easier for you to do squats with your own body weight, making exercise more pleasurable. Breathing exercises, relaxation, and the resulting ability to cope with stress will free up energies that would be otherwise wasted and dispersed by negative emotions such as anger, allowing you to redirect those energies toward achieving your goals.

Accomplishing your short-term goals will further inspire you to visualize your long-term goals. The self-knowledge you gain during the process will enable you to be more precise in detailing your long-term goals. (That is why I encourage you to wait until you have achieved at least some of your short-term goals before completing the part of the contract asking you to set one-year goals.) For example, if you can lose ten pounds in three months, it is reasonable to plan to lose twenty-five pounds in a year. (Avoid the trap of assuming that the initial pace of progress can be or should be maintained forever.) With a stronger and lighter body fuelled by wholesome food of better quality, you can set your sights more precisely on various improvements in lower-body, torso, and upper-body strength. With improved skills in coping with stress, you may also want to widen the scope of your training by participating in various recreational or competitive activities. These long-term goals can be revised and adjusted according to your rate of progress and health status.

One more thought: You may wish to finish your initial read-through of this book before attempting to set goals for your fitness program. That way, you will have a little more knowledge about the principles and terminology of the exercise program I recommend. For example, how can you set a goal to complete, say, twenty trunk curls if you don't even know what a trunk curl is?

Goal-Oriented Mindsets

As I mentioned before, goals encourage a positive attitude, and they provide us with stronger motivation, firmer commitment, better discipline, sharper focus, and enhanced patience and perseverance. But it is a two-way street, for besides inspiring these qualities, goals also rely on these qualities. The rest of the chapter discusses the reciprocal relationship between goals and the mindsets necessary to achieving them.

Positive Attitude

The ability to make an intelligent and consistent effort and the related ability to resist the temptation to give up are positive attitudes, both of which are inspired by having goals to work toward. Goals move us toward where we want to be and encourage us to go on. They help us overcome inertia and fear. Conversely, embracing a positive outlook—a belief that we can do what we set our minds to—also helps us achieve our goals.

Motivation

Motivation is our inner drive and the impulse that makes us act. It is the engine that gives us the mental and emotional energy we need to propel us forward. Some people lack motivation; they have no energy, momentum, inclination, or incentive to get going. As a result they are inactive or passive. Setting goals and visualizing yourself achieving them will help you get moving and will give you the impetus and energy to act.

Some people have a certain amount of drive, but that drive may be vague, dispersed, and misdirected. Blind drive is not conducive to success. Rather, it leads to frustration, failure, and defeat. *If we want to be successful our motivation needs commitment, focus, discipline, and direction—all of which can be fostered by setting realistic goals.* It is not enough to get excited and enthusiastic about something. Without motivation we would not be attracted to the idea of getting fit, but without serious commitment, discipline, and focus, motivation would fade rapidly.

Commitment

Commitment is the act of making up your mind, pledging yourself to a cause, embracing a course, and engaging yourself in a plan of action. Once we set our sights on a goal, we must make a commitment to take measured, decisive, and immediate action to achieve it. The longer you postpone committing yourself, the more you behave like the proverbial fisherman who decided to wait for the ocean to drain away so he could collect his fish. But the ocean (in this case, excuses) will be there forever.

With regard to physical training, commitment translates into the amount of time, effort, patience, persistence, discipline, and hard work you are prepared to dedicate toward achieving your goal. Commitment is among the most important strategies that increase your likelihood of success. It is the starting point for the realization of goals. During the process of achieving your goals, you must constantly foster, maintain, and increase your level of commitment, for it is the psychological foundation on which training, achievement, and success are built.

Discipline

Discipline is the glue that holds our thinking and actions together. Without discipline, neither our thinking nor our actions have organization, cohesion, direction, or focus. The term "discipline," which comes from the Latin word *disciplina,* means training for order, self-control, and efficiency of action according to a system of proven methods. *You will achieve your goals only if you follow the rules of training without compromise.* Any laxity (lack of care and concern) will make you a plaything of your mood and inclination. Your workouts will be irregular, your progression erratic, and the result will be failure and defeat.

Focus

Focus is the uninterrupted connection between you and whatever activity you are engaged in. It can make the difference in performing exercises correctly—that is, with good form, good posture, and good breathing. The ability to focus makes it possible to be absorbed in the movement, blocking out any distracting thoughts and emotions. The ability to seek, find, hold onto, and be absorbed in the feel of the movement adds quality to your exercises. If you lack focus, you just go through the motions without proper attention to coordination, range of motion, or fluidity of movement. The exercises you perform may make your muscles stronger, but if your technique lacks quality, any strength you gain will have little functional value.

Patience and Persistence

The ability to be patient and to persevere without losing interest or heart before things work out in your favor is absolutely necessary to achieving your goals. When working toward the goal of improving fitness through strength training, if you are impatient and want immediate results you will rush and fail to pay due attention to correct form, correct posture, correct breathing, and gradual progression. You will risk injury and burnout. Or you may observe the rules of training, but in your impatience to reach your goals you may exercise more frequently and with more intensity than your body is able to handle and adapt to. Although you may achieve your first goal sooner, your body will be unable to keep up with the demands imposed on it, and you will fail to achieve your long-term goals. Frustrated and defeated, you will lose heart before you can enjoy the benefits of your efforts. Setting realistic short-term and long-term goals and enjoying the process of achieving them will teach you how to be patient and persistent.

• • • • •

Goals can range from wanting to be able to climb stairs to wanting to be able to canoe down a river. Some people have a goal of getting into a dress of a certain size or looking good in a swimsuit. Whatever your fitness-related goals, use them to guide and energize your activities. The trick is to start with a pretty good idea of your present health and fitness status—your abilities and potentials—and then to establish goals that will serve as both challenge and roadmap.

Sample Exercise/Lifestyle Commitment Contract

I, _____Mighty Senior_____, pledge that

- I will do strength training three times a week on the following nonconsecutive days: _____Monday_____, _____Wednesday_____, and _____Friday_____.

- I will adhere to the appropriate guidelines for strength training, including proper warm-up, correct execution of exercises, stretching, and cool-down.

- I will walk briskly at least thirty minutes daily to improve and maintain my cardiovascular fitness, and I will practice breathing exercises twice a day.

- In order to maximize my improvements and to fully realize my potential, I will systematically improve my lifestyle habits in the areas of nutrition and stress management, practice breathing exercises twice a day, and give myself opportunities to relax.

- My short-term goals for the next three months are the following:
  - a. Lose _____10_____ lbs.
  - b. Be able to _____complete a set of 12 half-squats_____
  - c. Be able to _____complete a set of 12 wall push-ups_____

- My long-term goals for the year are the following:

  - a. Lose _____30_____ lbs.
  - b. Lower my blood pressure to _____normal_____
  - c. Be able to _complete a set of 12 half squats with 10-lb. dumbells_
  - d. Be able to _complete a set of 12 bench presses with 15 lb. dumbells_
  - e. Be able to _hike for two hours on a trail_

- I will keep a daily record of my activities.

- Every day I will reaffirm my commitment to doing all of the above.

- I will find ways of rewarding myself for every improvement.

_____Mighty Senior_____   _April 21, 2006_

SIGNATURE   DATE

Exercise/Lifestyle Commitment Contract

I, _____, pledge that

- I will do strength training three times a week on the following nonconsecutive days: _____, _____, and _____.

- I will adhere to the appropriate guidelines for strength training, including proper warm-up, correct execution of exercises, stretching, and cool-down.

- I will walk briskly at least thirty minutes daily to improve and maintain my cardiovascular fitness, and I will practice breathing exercises twice a day.

- In order to maximize my improvements and to fully realize my potential, I will systematically improve my lifestyle habits in the areas of nutrition and stress management, practice breathing exercises twice a day, and give myself opportunities to relax.

- My short-term goals for the next three months are the following:
  a. Lose _____ lbs.
  b. Be able to _____
  c. Be able to _____

- My long-term goals for the year are the following:
  a. Lose _____ lbs.
  b. Lower my blood pressure to _____
  c. Be able to _____
  d. Be able to _____
  e. Be able to _____

- I will keep a daily record of my activities.

- Every day I will reaffirm my commitment to doing all of the above.

- I will find ways of rewarding myself for every improvement.

_____   _____

SIGNATURE   DATE

6 | Principles of Strength Training for Seniors

You will probably experience some level of improvement in your strength by following almost any strength-training program, but unless the program meets certain fundamental principles, your gains will be erratic and short-lived. Some popular programs can result in spectacular short-term gains, but they carry a high risk of injury and burnout. The increased strength they afford is usually unbalanced and almost never translates into functional skill. Other popular programs are too generalized to be effective and thus fail to provide a reasonable rate of improvement.

To meet our requirements, a well-designed training program for seniors must be

1. *Safe:* It must be designed and executed to minimize the potential for injury and the likelihood of aggravating existing medical conditions or creating new ones.
2. *Effective:* It must be designed, executed, and constantly adjusted so that it produces the best possible results. It must remain both challenging and stimulating without straining the body. The frequency, intensity, and complexity of the workouts must be manipulated so that the result will be a steady and optimal gain in muscle strength. Appropriate periods of rest (recovery) and consolidation must be built in. (Consolidation occurs when the exerciser slows down or ceases progression to allow him or her to firmly establish the results achieved so far.)
3. *Personalized:* It must take into account the specific needs of the individual, such as health and fitness status, biological age, potential for gain, and short- and long-term goals.
4. *Functional:* It must translate the improvements in muscle strength into real-life, functional capabilities.
5. *Progressive:* It must ensure progress toward your goals. Once certain gains have been achieved and firmly established, further

improvements are targeted. There is always something to be improved—from coordination to posture, from flexibility to muscle endurance.

6. *Balanced:* It must develop the musculature in a balanced and proportionate manner. It must also balance several other aspects of fitness, including posture, flexibility, and gait.

Let's look at each of these principles in more detail.

Safe

You have acquainted yourself with the basics of human anatomy, and with the location and workings of your musculature. After careful consideration, you will design your initial training program based on your medical history, fitness assessment, biological age, and activity level. You will take into account the level of your physical skills, including coordination, reaction time, sense of balance, and speed of movement. Finding the optimal exercises, the optimal workload, and the optimal rate of progression will still occur by trial and error. Injuries and the possibility of aggravating existing medical conditions or creating new ones not only can stop you from continuing training but may also seriously affect your health, so it is wise to be cautious when you embark on your strength-training program.

The goal is for your body to respond to strength training with a series of positive adaptations—not aggravations. To design a safe program you will select the exercises; determine the frequency, intensity, and duration of training sessions; choose the level of resistance (amount of weight); and set the pace of progression with this objective in mind.

Exercise Selection

You can choose from a wide range of strength-training exercises involving various degrees of difficulty and complexity. *If you start strength training after a long period of inactivity and your level of strength fitness is fairly low, it is wise to select simple and relatively easy exercises for your initial program.* Increase the level of your strength and skills with these simple and less demanding exercises in a patient and gradual manner. *Progress toward more complicated and difficult exercises only after your gains are consolidated and confirmed.*

For example, for beginners with low strength and skill levels, it is wise to initially choose wall push-ups (also called push-aways); leave regular push-ups for later. Exercise your legs by standing up from a bench; postpone squats for when your leg strength and sense of balance improve. Beginners should also avoid overhead movements with weights and exercises that involve countermovements, such as lunges. Generally speaking, always stay within your comfort level, and always make sure that the exercises you choose do not strain your body or overextend your abilities.

Frequency of Workouts

Always remember that exercise stresses your tissues, causing microscopic damage to your muscles, tendons, and ligaments. Stressed tissues must undergo a repair and rebuilding process that may last for forty-eight to ninety-six hours. If you give your body the necessary time to repair and rebuild itself, you will steadily improve your strength fitness. On the other hand, if you do a workout before the repair and rebuilding processes are completed, your tissues will slowly degrade, but if you wait too long until the next workout, your body will have passed the optimal period of readiness and you will experience little or no progress (the "use it or lose it" principle).

I find that *two or three training sessions per week on nonconsecutive days is the optimal frequency for strength training.* To make sure the body's recovery is complete, I like to train the lower body and torso in one session and the upper body and torso in the next. The muscles of the torso—because of the lack of joints, tendons, and ligaments and because of the proximity to large blood vessels—tend to recover faster than muscles in other parts of the body.

Intensity of Workouts

Intensity is the amount of work done within a certain period. The more work you compress into a workout, the heavier the resistance you use, the faster your movements are, and the less rest you take between sets and exercises, the more intense your workouts are.

I recommend that when seniors embark on a strength-training program they *keep the intensity of their workouts between low and moderate.* By this I mean exercising against low to moderate resistance, performing the movements slowly, and taking plenty of rest between sets of exercises. The time between sets and between various exercises should be used for stretching, breathing, and visualizing (mentally rehearsing) the next exercise or set.

Duration of Workouts

Depending on the health, fitness status, and biological age of the person, the duration of each strength-training session can be between twenty and sixty minutes. *It is safer to start with shorter sessions and gradually increase workout time as you progress.*

Resistance

Resistance, be it from gravity or an elastic band, is the opposing force pitted against the force of your muscles in action. Your muscles may defeat that force (concentric muscle action), may hold a contraction against it without producing any movement (isometric muscle action), or may have to yield to it while trying to resist it (eccentric muscle action). In my opinion, seniors should avoid exercises requiring both isometric and eccentric actions. This means the strength-training exercises we select should employ only concentric muscle action.

What is the best way of determining the optimal resistance you want to tackle to exercise your muscles? If I say that you should exercise your muscles against a force that is about 75 percent of the maximum force you can produce, I might tempt you to test your maximum strength, and no senior should ever do that. *The best and safest way of determining optimal resistance is to perform a particular exercise and adjust the resistance until you find that you can execute the movement eight to twelve times (eight to twelve repetitions) without straining and while maintaining correct form, proper posture, and a proper breathing pattern.*

Three sets of eight to twelve repetitions with two or three minutes of rest between each set is a good protocol to follow to achieve optimal strength gains safely and effectively.

Pace of Progression

Progression is the movement in the direction of your goals. My most important observation in training myself and in training and observing others is that *rushing progression actually hinders it.* Whenever you increase the rate and pace of progression above what is optimal, you not only risk injuries, plateaus, burnouts, and maladaptations (negative responses), but you also upset the body's rhythm and cycle of absorbing stress and repairing and rebuilding tissue by imposing more stress on it through heavier workloads. The result can be physically and psychologically devastating.

It is very important to exercise prudence and patience and to *plan progression so that your workouts challenge your body without aggravating it.*

At the beginning, newcomers to strength training usually experience improvements that are quite spectacular. It is normal to experience a 50 to 75 percent increase in one's strength during the first couple of months of training. However, this initial increase in ability to perform more work is due mostly to neural rather than anatomical adaptations. This means that although there is very little improvement in the strength of the individual muscles and muscle fibers, you still become able to perform more work because your central nervous system learns how to organize, coordinate, and recruit your individual muscles and muscle fibers more efficiently. Your physical resources remain about the same, but your nervous system, through more efficient processing and more effective control mechanisms, is able to get more work out of your muscles.

It is a mistake to think that this fast initial rate of progress will be permanent. How, then, do you determine your optimal rate of progression over the medium and long term?

Set the initial resistance at a level against which you can perform a particular exercise eight to twelve times. Make sure you perform the exercise correctly, with proper posture and breathing (described in Chapter 7). When you are able to correctly perform sixteen repetitions of the same exercise in three sets without overextending and straining yourself, spend a week establishing these strength gains, during which time you focus on improving all aspects of your form. After this week of consolidation, once again increase the resistance so that you can perform the same exercise only eight to twelve times while maintaining correct form and without straining yourself.

Later in your progress there will be a limit to how much you can increase the level of resistance. It is a common mistake and a source of possible injuries and disappointments to measure improvements solely by the amount of work you are able to perform (i.e., how much weight you can use). Other, equally important aspects of improvement are reflected in qualitative changes, such as an increase in skill level, postural improvement, and better gait. Because there is a limit to the amount of force you will be able to generate, a simple-minded preoccupation with being able to work against heavier and heavier resistance will limit your prospects. At the same time, there is almost no end to learning and refining your skills. Rather than focusing solely on how much resistance you can work against, I highly recommend widening the scope of your aspirations to include

- perfecting your form and technical skills
- increasing the variety of exercises
- increasing the level of complexity of the exercises
- introducing new training modalities into your program, such as various recreational and competitive activities (e.g., canoeing, kayaking, hiking, swimming, aerobic dance, yoga, Pilates)

Other Considerations

Although later chapters deal more fully with proper warm-up and cooldown, and with performing exercises in their full range of motion, I want to touch on these considerations as part of the discussion of safety.

A warm-up—that is, a gradual increase in the body's activity level—is a very important way of avoiding injury. Good warm-ups improve circulation (safely elevating heart rate and expanding the walls of blood vessels), lead to more efficient metabolism (elevating the intensity of transport of nutrients to the working muscles and enhancing the removal of waste products), increase body awareness, refresh muscle memory, and raise the level of preparedness of the bodily systems so that they will be better able to meet the demands of strength training.

At the end of the workout, a *cool-down, by allowing your bodily systems to slowly lower the level of intensity of their operations, ensures a smooth transition from an active to less active state.* This will help avoid aggravations that may happen if you abruptly end your work out.

When exercisers and trainers talk about the importance of a full range of motion, some fail to mention that "full" is a relative term. Every individual has a different level of joint mobility. Furthermore, a person's mobility level may vary from time to time, from one exercise to the other, and according to the level of resistance involved in a particular exercise. *You should never force your joints to move beyond a pain-free range of motion.* Always stay within your comfort level to avoid straining your joints. Go to the point of pain, but never through pain.

Effective

An effective program or procedure consistently produces the best possible results. Our discussion of the various requirements of safe exercising already addressed some aspects of effective training. Here I'll deal only with the ability to produce the best results consistently.

An effective training program will bring out the best in your body. *It will elicit maximum gains and help you reach your maximum potential* without losing sight of safety and without stepping over the boundaries of prudence and reason. It will provide optimal stimulus and challenge for your body. If the level, quality, and nature of the stimuli are just about right at the beginning of your program and are progressively adjusted as your strength fitness improves, you will achieve your maximum potential.

To determine the most effective way of improving your strength fitness, you must consider every aspect of your health and fitness, your biological age, your level of activity, and your goals. For example, although table tennis and bowling may improve your muscle speed and coordination, neither is an effective way of improving your strength fitness. Nor is physical labor an effective form of strength training, whether it involves low-intensity activities such as gardening or higher-intensity activities such as plastering a wall. Working out with a balance board or an exercise ball and doing yoga and breathing exercises are effective ways of improving posture, flexibility, range of motion, balance, coordination, movement skills, and functional abilities, but they are not in and of themselves sufficient for strength training. In my opinion, as I've said, an ideal exercise regimen should address all these aspects of fitness.

It has been proven that the most effective way of improving one's strength fitness is through resistance training, but resistance training must meet certain requirements to be effective. If we use a resistance that is too low to stimulate our muscles, or if we use the same monotonous routine each time we train, we will fail to achieve our maximum potential. For the muscles to become as strong as they can be, our strength-training program must be physically and mentally challenging and stimulating, and it must be varied regularly. It must provide the optimal maximum impact on the muscles to which they can respond positively.

Personalized

One of the basic problems with most popular programs is that while they may satisfy the general needs of an arbitrarily established statistical average, they fail to address the specific needs and goals of the individual. *It is very important that a strength-training program be designed and executed to fit the individual's needs rather than the individual trying to fit the program.* The program must be designed, reassessed, and adjusted to suit the person—not the other way around.

It is always the program that fails the individual. The individual should never feel obliged to adjust his or her aspirations or to override personal and specific health and fitness concerns in order to satisfy the prescriptions of any program.

When someone forces his or her various bodily systems to absorb and adapt to a program that is not designed to meet his or her individual needs, the following *physical* maladaptations (negative responses) can occur:

- Acute and chronic injuries and illnesses
- Muscle imbalance
- Lack of gains in strength
- Lack of maintainable progress

The following detrimental *psychological* effects can also occur:

- Low self-esteem resulting from a perception that one is not good enough to execute the program
- Frustration resulting from lack of positive stimuli and positive response
- Generally negative feelings toward exercise, resulting in lack of enjoyment and satisfaction and, finally, in quitting the exercise program

It is very important to design a personalized program by acquainting yourself with the basics of strength training and by learning as much as you can about the state of your health and fitness. You must also constantly reassess and readjust your program to your changing needs. A personalized program, which will evolve by thoughtful planning as much as by trial and error, will fit your specific needs and will move you toward your goals safely and effectively. Developing a personalized program will be more mentally demanding than simply adopting a generalized program, but your efforts will be rewarded. You will

- learn more about yourself, your abilities, and your potential during the process
- have the satisfaction of taking responsibility and independent action
- enjoy a sense of empowerment through defining your goals and aspirations
- be an active and informed participant in planning, assessing, and shaping your program (even if some of it is done in consultation with a fitness professional)
- achieve better results

Initially it is helpful to consult a qualified fitness professional. This investment may save you from frustrations that can result from unproductive and misdirected efforts.

Functional

Your exercise program must be functional, which means that *gains in strength must be translated into real-life abilities*. The muscle-by-muscle, exercise-by-exercise interpretation of muscle strength can be misleading. As a result, some exercisers work their muscles in isolation, completely disregarding the fact that the practical usefulness of muscle strength gained in such a manner is usually quite small. You may improve the ability of the triceps to extend your arm against resistance, and you may also improve the ability of the biceps to flex your arm more powerfully, but if your exercises focus on only one or two muscle groups, with very little or no involvement from the rest of your body, the strength you gain will not be fully functional.

The long-term goal of improving your strength is not to enable you to do more biceps curls, squats, and abdominal curls, but to make sure that you enjoy life through physical independence and the ability to participate in various satisfying physical activities. To gain muscle strength is a good short-term goal, but the long-term goal is to have strength that improves your quality of life, not just that of your individual muscles.

How do we transform the extra strength your muscles gain into more powerful real-life movement and the ability to participate in real-life activities? One way is to gradually widen the range of exercises so that they involve more and more muscles. As your overall strength increases, you can add to your program more difficult and more complex exercises that require the coordinated participation of your whole body. Another way of achieving functional strength is to perform the exercises in ways that resemble real-life demands and situations requiring balance, agility, and various other skills. Instead of performing certain exercises on a bench, you can do them on an exercise ball. At a certain point you may want to participate in various recreational or competitive activities, such as hiking, swimming, playing tennis, or canoeing.

Progressive

Progression is the process of moving in the direction of your goals. Depending on your genetics, biological age, health, and fitness status, you have a certain strength potential. The realization of this potential is one of your long-term goals. Using progressive strength-training methods, you will be able to move toward this goal.

Strength has many aspects, including the following:

- *Maximum strength,* which is measured by the maximum resistance you are able to defeat
- *Relative strength,* which is your strength measured relative to your body weight
- *Strength endurance,* which is your ability to repeatedly defeat resistance for a prolonged period
- *Functional strength,* which is the strength needed to perform real-life tasks

While progressions in maximum strength and relative strength are valid goals and are certainly the easiest to measure, I discourage seniors from focusing solely on improving these aspects of strength. In fact, I strongly recommend that you avoid testing your maximum or relative strength.

To achieve progress in every aspect of your strength fitness, your program must include the following:

- A progressive and gradual increase in the resistance your muscles must defeat (interspersed with periods of consolidation)
- A progressive increase in the variety of exercises
- A progressive increase in the difficulty and complexity of exercises and activities

Balanced

A balanced strength-training program will ensure that *the whole musculature of your body is improved proportionately.* If we widen the concept of balance to include all aspects of fitness, we mean that every important component of your fitness is properly considered and improved in a balanced manner. You may have a certain bias for a particular aspect of fitness (such as strength), but you should not disregard other important components, such as flexibility.

• • • • •

The next chapter discusses the proper elements that should be included in every strength-training session.

7 | Your Strength-Training Routine
Elements to Include in Every Exercise Session

To be successful in any endeavor, we need an effective working method, a systematic procedure for getting results.[1] *It is very important to follow a proper and well-established routine during your strength-training sessions.* Each exercise has its own special pattern of correct execution, for which you will find detailed instructions in the chapters devoted to describing the exercises. This chapter deals with a bigger picture: the fundamental elements that must be included in each strength-training session. Regardless of the specific exercises you're doing, each session must follow certain general guidelines, including the following:

- Preparations for a safe training environment
- Physical and mental/emotional warm-up
- Establishing and maintaining proper posture
- Executing movements slowly and in a controlled manner
- Aiming for a full range of motion
- Establishing and maintaining a breathing pattern of regular, deep inhalations and full exhalations
- Generating positive feelings related to the movements
- Performing exercises in a specific order
- Cool-down
- Stretching

Let's take a closer look at each of these guidelines.

Preparations for a Safe Training Environment

To ensure that accidents will not happen, before each training session you must make sure that your immediate surroundings are safe. Check that

- the floor is free of objects that may cause you to trip

1. M. Fekete, "The Role of Continuing Education in the NSCA," *Strength and Conditioning* 21, no. 4 (1999): 67–70.

- there are no obstructions within your range that would interfere with your movements
- pieces of equipment are orderly, stacked, and secured
- your equipment, training attire, and shoes are safe and in good working order

Whether you are training in a club or at home, with machines or with free weights, it is very important that you observe and follow the rules of safety regarding exercise equipment and attire. Everything—from your shoes and shoelaces to the plates on your dumbbell—must be examined to make sure that accidents will not happen. Even if you have a safe and effective training program and know how to perform the exercises well, you can still risk injuries through neglect and lack of care. A plate that isn't secured properly may fall off the barbell, or you can trip over a dumbbell left on the floor. Resulting injuries may set you back for months. Performing a routine visual and manual check of the training area and equipment before each session will substantially reduce your risk of injuries by ensuring that you avoid silly and annoying accidents.

As you perform your check, watch for the following:

- Benches must sit firmly on the floor, plates must be secured properly on barbells and dumbbells (I have seen loose plates fall off and cause serious injury), and machines must be correctly loaded and set.
- Always remove unneeded equipment from the area where you exercise. Always stack unused dumbbells on a rack. Even towels, your water bottle, and other miscellaneous items should be placed out of the way so that you will not slip, trip, or fall over them.
- Always make sure that no one in your close proximity is performing exercises, such as overhead lifts, that could lead to injury if the person drops the weight, loses his or her balance, or falls.
- Even little things, such as ensuring that your shoelaces are properly tied, may prevent an accident. Your clothes should fit well so they will not hinder movements or get caught on equipment.
- Always have a towel handy so you can wipe the sweat off your face (to keep it from dripping into your eyes and causing visual obstruction) and hands (so your hands won't slip when you're handling heavy equipment).

Physical and Mental/Emotional Warm-Up

It is very important that you physically and mentally warm up before performing exercises. *Physical warm-up is absolutely necessary to make sure that your body reacts positively to exercise.* Any sudden effort may strain your heart and could adversely affect every system, from arteries to joints to muscles to central nervous system. When you're at rest, your various bodily systems operate at a relatively low level of intensity and readiness. Your heart beats at a resting heart rate, and the diameter of your arteries is calibrated for a normal flow of blood. The release of various enzymes and hormones is slowed. Your joints are not lubricated, and your metabolism, including the transport of nutrients and the processing and removal of waste products, is idling. Your senses are less finely tuned, and your resulting perception may be less sharp than it should be.

As we age, warming up becomes even more important because the walls of our arteries are stiffer and need more time to expand to accommodate an increased volume of blood. Our joints are dehydrated and need longer to be lubricated by synovial fluid. Our senses and reflexes are slower and need some practice to become alert and to respond promptly.

At the beginning of each training session, gently warm up by doing the following activities:

- Perform rhythmical movements, such as walking on a treadmill or walking in place. Make sure that your posture is correct and expresses confidence and vitality, that your gait has bounce and energy, and that your breathing is efficient. (See below for more about proper posture and breathing.)
- Execute movements slowly, concentrating on coordination and precision.
- Tense and relax your muscles rhythmically.
- Do some breathing exercises as described in Chapter 4, focusing on deep inhalations and full exhalations.

Figures 7.1 through 7.5, on the next two pages, illustrate some good warm-up moves. After doing a general warm-up, it is a good idea before each exercise to perform the movements of that particular exercise a few times without added resistance. Warming up in this way helps you practice correct form, correct posture, and correct breathing. It also refreshes muscle memory as you activate the prime movers that will execute the same exercise against resistance.

It is also a good idea to go through a mental/emotional rehearsal before beginning your workout. *Establishing a positive mindset at the beginning of each session and maintaining it throughout the whole session is just as important as warming up physically.* View your warm-up as preparing you for something good, something enjoyable. Warming up involves more than moving certain body parts. It involves more than elevating body temperature and heart rate. It is almost a ceremonial act of elevating your mood and consciousness. Here are some tips to help you mentally warm up for your workout:

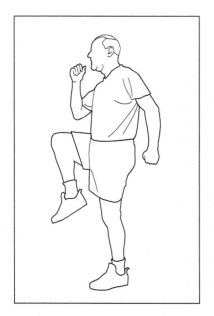

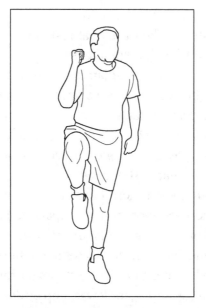

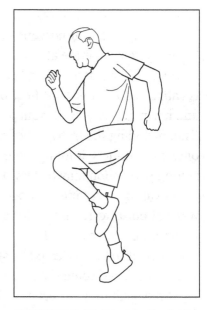

FIGURE 7.1A. *Walking in place with knee lift and elbow drive — Side view*

FIGURE 7.1B. *Walking in place with knee lift and elbow drive — Front view*

FIGURE 7.2. *Walking on the balls of the feet*

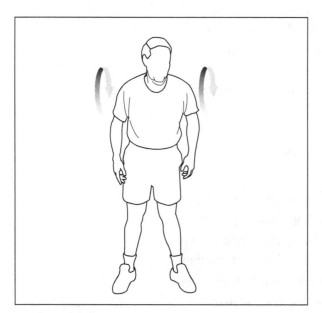

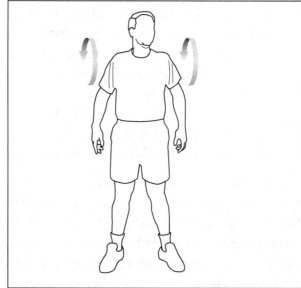

FIGURE 7.3A. *Rotating the shoulders forward*

FIGURE 7.3B. *Rotating the shoulders backward*

- Imagine yourself moving with energy and confidence.
- Visualize yourself performing the exercises with fluid, coordinated, and precise motions.
- Produce positive emotions by thinking of your exercise session as an important step in your progress toward your goals.

For more about generating positive feelings toward exercise in general, also see the related section below.

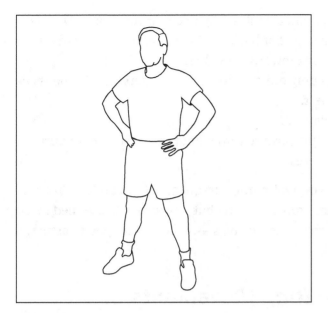

FIGURE 7.4A. *Standing good morning — Starting position*

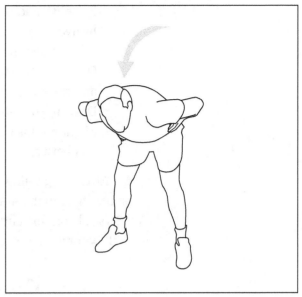

FIGURE 7.4B. *Standing good morning — Finishing position*

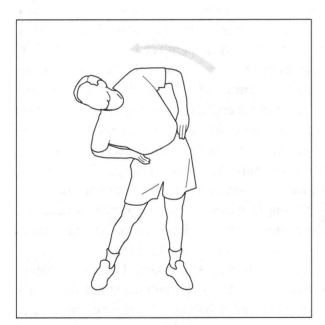

FIGURE 7.5A. *Tilting the trunk toward the left*

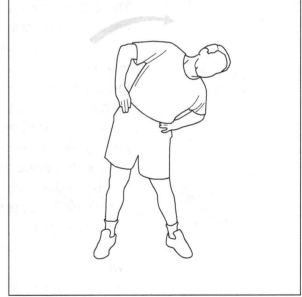

FIGURE 7.5B. *Tilting the trunk toward the right*

Maintaining Proper Posture

Correct posture is one of the most important aspects of physical fitness. Along with strength, good posture helps to improve one's mental and emotional well-being. Although each exercise calls for its own specific posture, there are general guidelines for regulating the way we stand, sit, and carry ourselves. At the beginning of each training session, adjust and align the various parts of your body by going through the following steps:

- Establish and maintain a neutral alignment in your spine. Do this by avoiding hunching your back, pushing your head forward, or letting your chin sink toward your chest.
- Once you are standing erect, draw your shoulders a bit farther back and raise your chest.
- Draw in your stomach.
- Maintain this healthy posture throughout the session, both during and between exercises.

At the beginning, you will require frequent self-reminders and constant effort to maintain proper posture, but as you get accustomed to the physical comfort and the better feelings associated with good posture, it will become automatic.

Executing Movements at the Proper Speed

It is important to perform the exercises slowly and in a controlled manner. There are several reasons why this is true. If you move too fast, the distribution of work through the range of movement becomes uneven. To create speed you preload (overload) the muscles at the beginning of the motion, and the resulting momentum will almost carry the movement through the remaining part of the exercise without requiring much effort from your muscles. By contrast, using slow and controlled movements allows you to distribute force production evenly among the various motor units of your individual muscles through the entire range of motion.

Fast movements also lead to abrupt rebounding from one end of the motion to the other, resulting in sudden countermovements that may strain your joints, tendons, and ligaments. Slow and controlled motions are more forgiving for your joints, tendons, and ligaments.

You can use your breathing pattern to set the pace of your movements. (We will deal in detail with proper breathing pattern later.) Follow the rhythm of deep inhalations and full exhalations to regulate movement speed. If you make sure that you lower the weight in synch with your full inhalation and raise it in tandem with your full exhalation, you cannot go wrong with movement speed.

Aiming for a Full Range of Motion

In strength training it is important to perform exercises in their full range of movement. This means starting the movement with a full muscle stretch and completing it with a full muscle contraction. We do this for the following two reasons:

1. to develop a full range of muscle strength at every angle of the motion
2. to develop full joint flexibility

However, you must keep in mind that developing a full range of movement is a long-term goal, especially for exercisers who have various conditions that restrict range of movement or who start strength training after a long period of inactivity. Biological age also contributes to muscle and joint stiffness.

Furthermore, although your goal is to achieve a full range of motion, it is also very important never to move beyond a pain-free range of motion. Forcing your joints, muscles, tendons, and ligaments to do something they are incapable of doing will inevitably lead to injuries. If necessary, you must also eliminate exercises that cause immediate or delayed pain in your joints. Exercising steadily and consistently and keeping your movements within a safe and comfortable range will gradually extend your range of motion.

Maintaining Proper Breathing

Although I give specific breathing instructions for each exercise, there are a few general rules that must be followed regardless of the particular exercise you're doing.

Do not hold your breath while exercising. You must breathe continuously throughout each repetition of every exercise. Holding your breath while making an effort may produce excessive internal pressure that, in turn, can restrict the flow of blood through your veins (the vessels that transport blood back to the heart). Restricted blood flow can cause both pooling of blood in the veins and high blood pressure, possibly resulting in symptoms such as dizziness and light-headedness. These can result in temporary loss of control of your muscles.

Regulate your breathing. Random breathing—breathing that is out of synch with the rhythm of your movements—can be just as bad as holding your breath. Fast breathing may cause hyperventilation, may be distracting, and may reduce your ability to exercise control over technique and form. The general rule for how to regulate your breathing is to exhale as you overcome the resistance (positive phase), and inhale as you yield to the resistance (negative phase). This pattern allows the contracted muscles to stretch and get ready for the next positive phase. Let us say, for example, that you are performing a wall push-up. Inhale when you move toward the wall, and exhale when you push away from the wall.

There are a few exceptions to this general rule. When you're doing a biceps curl or a one-arm row, some fitness books and some trainers recommend that you inhale during the positive phase. In these exercises the positive effort is made during the movement toward (rather than away from) the body. That means you're defeating resistance as you pull. The expansion of the chest that results from a full inhalation during a pulling movement provides a solid platform and ensures correct posture for the exercise. You can practice one and then the other pattern of breathing while performing these exercises to see which pattern is more suitable for you. If you think doing this will be confusing, stick to the general rule of exhaling through the positive phase (i.e., while overcoming the resistance) and inhaling through the negative phase (i.e., while yielding to the resistance).

As already mentioned, it is important to both inhale and exhale fully and slowly, and to do so in synch with the two movement phases of each exercise. Shallow breaths provide insufficient oxygen to the lungs, reduce the calming effect of slow and deep breathing, and break up the rhythm of movement as well as the synch between movement and breathing.

Generating Positive Feelings Related to Exercise

It is important to generate positive feelings and sensations as you exercise. Otherwise, exercise becomes a chore or a duty, and you end up performing the movements like a robot. In fact, exercise becomes an added stress. Positive feelings and intellectual awareness of what you're doing mutually enhance each other and make exercising a satisfying experience.

Positive feelings and sensations act as the driving force behind the knowledge that exercise is good for you. They add enjoyment to each movement and to each inhalation and exhalation. They help release endorphins into the bloodstream that, in turn, further increase the joy and pleasure of exercise. You can double the value of each session by generating and maintaining positive emotions while exercising.

Here are a few practical tips for how to produce positive feelings about exercise:

- Enjoy the rhythm of breathing and movement. Be proud of your ability to find your own rhythm.
- Enjoy the good effort you are making. Whenever you sense the negative feeling of resistance bearing down on your muscles, turn it around immediately and feel the force of your muscles defeating that resistance. Take pleasure in this satisfying feeling.
- Visualize and feel your lungs expanding as you inhale fresh air, and feel the good work your heart does in pumping fresh blood to the working muscles and the lungs.
- Enjoy being in your element when you are exercising.

Performing Exercises in an Appropriate Order

After you warm up, start with exercises that involve the larger muscle groups. Leave the smaller muscles for last.

For balanced muscle development, whenever possible pair exercises so that opposing muscle groups are exercised one right after the other. For example, after exercising the chest muscles, exercise the muscles of the upper back. After exercising the triceps, exercise the biceps, and so on. Some exercises simultaneously exercise opposing muscle groups, such as the squat, which exercises both the quadriceps and the hamstrings.

Cool-Down

A sudden and abrupt cessation of exercise may strain the heart. For this reason it is highly recommended that, after your regular exercises, you perform certain rhythmical movements, such as walking in place. As you cool down, make sure to continue practicing correct posture and to inhale and exhale regularly and deeply. These rhythmical movements, done without resistance, serve to gradually wind down your strength-training session, helping you to transition smoothly from a higher-than-normal level of intensity to your usual degree of functioning.

Stretching

You should both stretch your working muscles after each set and stretch your whole body after your cool-down. Stretching must be gentle and should be done so that you never strain your joints. Especially avoid straining your back. Refer to page 105 for basic stretching exercises.

• • • • •

The next chapter will help you use everything you've learned so far as you create your initial strength-training program.

8 | Designing Your Initial Program

Knowing the basic principles of training and the elements that must be included in every workout session will provide you with a good foundation for designing a strength-training program. Now let's imagine a few scenarios that will allow us to put the knowledge base we have built to practical use. In this chapter I outline two examples of strength-training programs, each based on various hypothetical medical and fitness parameters. You will see that whatever your health and fitness status, and whatever your biological age, there is no reason to postpone your goal of gaining strength and reaping all the rewards that come with it.

It is a good idea to keep a record of your strength-training sessions. This way, you can both chronicle your progress (because you are rewarding yourself in some way for each step toward your goals) and review what you've been doing when the time comes to modify your program. I have included blank charts for this purpose in the back of the book. You can either cut them out of the book or photocopy them and use them to design your own programs. Sample charts are included in this chapter after each program description. Use them as a guide for how to complete the blank charts.

Important note: Seniors who have been inactive for most of their adult lives, who have poor balance, who are obese, or who otherwise lack sufficient muscle strength to perform some of the more strenuous exercises recommended here should start with a series of beginner exercises. These are described in the next chapter.

Program #1: Low Fitness Level Plus a Medical Condition

Let's say that you are a typical senior who has been cleared by your doctor for strength training. You have high blood pressure, have arthritis in the hips and knees, and are overweight by about twenty-five pounds. The combination of arthritis and excess weight makes it difficult for you to get up from a sitting position. You have been sedentary for the last ten years. Your chronological age is sixty, but the effects of bad lifestyle habits, inactivity, and the medical conditions of high blood pressure and arthritis put your biological age closer to sixty-seven.

You have already made up your mind to become physically active. You have started working on your lifestyle habits and have made significant changes in the right direction. You have also taken the first step toward getting more exercise by walking for twenty minutes each day before dinner.

It would make sense initially to plan two strength-training sessions per week, allowing two or three days of rest between sessions. As described in Chapter 6, train the lower body and torso in one session, and the upper body and torso in the next session. Later, when your fitness improves, you may want to increase the frequency of your strength-training workouts to three sessions per week. It would also make good sense to exercise for fifteen to twenty minutes in each session. Once your body consistently responds well to strength training for a full month, consider gradually increasing the duration of each session.

Because of your high blood pressure, your long history of inactivity, and your resulting biological age, you should start your strength training with very simple exercises, such as those described in the next chapter. You should also avoid the risks presented by high blood pressure by doing only those exercises that are performed in the upright position, such as sitting leg raises (page 83) or wall quarter squats performed against minimal resistance (described below). When the combined effects of good lifestyle habits, walking, and strength-training lower your weight and blood pressure, you can then add exercises that require positions other than an upright one, such as lying leg raises (page 84) or lying leg abductions (page 84).

Both your legs and upper body are relatively weak. Your arthritis and your extra weight make every exercise more difficult to perform. Considering everything, it is reasonable to suggest that, initially, you should do only two exercises for the legs, three exercises for the upper body, and one for the abs.

Lower-Body/Torso Program

1. Start with a warm-up, as described in Chapter 7. Walk in place for a few minutes while maintaining correct posture and doing deep inhalations and full exhalations.
2. For your first leg exercise, you can do sitting leg raises (page 83) or wall quarter squats. To do wall quarter squats, face the wall,

lean your hands against it at shoulder height, and place your legs about shoulder width apart. Bend (flex) your knees about twenty-five degrees, then straighten (extend) them. Inhale as you bend your knees, and exhale as you straighten them. Do three sets of eight to twelve repetitions, with two minutes of active rest between sets. (If you're doing sitting leg raises, do three sets of eight to twelve repetitions for each leg.) Active rest means walking in place while practicing deep inhalations and full exhalations.

3. The next leg exercise is standing leg abductions (page 92). Do three sets of eight to twelve repetitions for each leg, with two minutes of active rest between sets. At the beginning you will find that it is difficult to raise your leg more than fifteen to twenty degrees. You should avoid forcing your range of motion beyond what you are comfortable with.

4. With high blood pressure, you should not do abdominal crunches while lying on the floor, at least not until the combined effects of good lifestyle habits, walking, strength training, and deep breathing lower your blood pressure. The safest abdominal exercise for someone with your health and fitness status is the sitting knee raise (page 81). Do three sets of eight to twelve repetitions for each leg, with two minutes of active rest between sets. In a few weeks you may want to increase the difficulty of the exercise. Do so by placing your chair close enough to a table so that you can comfortably reach the tabletop with your hands to support yourself while you slowly raise *both* bent knees toward your chest.

5. For a cool-down, repeat your warm-up of walking in place while maintaining correct posture and while breathing with deep inhalations and full exhalations.

In a few weeks, as your legs and abs get stronger, you can increase the number of reps you do in each set to fourteen or sixteen. You can also add more advanced exercises, such as heel raises (page 91). You can switch from quarter to half squats. To do wall half squats, follow the instructions as above for wall quarter squats, but bend your knees more deeply.

Upper-Body/Torso Program

For upper-body exercises you can start with wall push-ups (described below) and biceps curls (page 104). Later, as your fitness improves, you can add other exercises, such as lateral arm raises (page 103).

1. Do your usual warm-up of walking in place and practicing deep inhalations and full exhalations.

2. Start with wall push-ups. Stand facing a wall, just far enough away so that your extended arms can reach the wall at shoulder

height and a little wider than shoulder width. Lean against the wall by slightly bending your elbows. Exhale to prepare for your first repetition. Now, inhale as you bend your elbows and lean toward the wall. Bend your elbows only as much as you feel comfortable with. Stop. Slowly push yourself away from the wall as you exhale. Perform eight to twelve repetitions in three sets with two minutes of active rest between sets.

3. The next exercise is biceps curls (page 104), which you can do standing, either away from the wall or with your back against a wall. Use weights of 2.5 to 5 pounds in each hand. Perform three sets of eight to twelve repetitions, with two minutes of active rest between sets. For active rest when you're doing upper-body work, put your weights down, then rotate your shoulders back and forth with your arms hanging by your side. Keep doing deep inhalations and full exhalations.

4. Next, do lateral arm raises. Do them as described on page 103, but in the beginning *do them without holding any weights*. (If you prefer, you can do sitting arm abductions, page 82, which are similar.) Do three sets of eight to twelve reps, with two minutes of active rest (shoulder rotations and deep breathing) between sets. Later, as your deltoid muscles become stronger, you can perform this exercise with a 1.5-pound dumbbell.

5. Continue with your abdominal exercises, which will be the same as the ones you did after your leg routine.

6. End your session with five minutes of cool-down, consisting of walking in place while maintaining good posture. Repeat the biceps curls without weights a few times, and practice deep inhalations and full exhalations.

In a few weeks, as your upper body gets stronger, you can add more advanced exercises, such as one-arm rowing (page 100), to this routine. Start by using a dumbbell weighing 5 to 10 pounds.

Program #1 (Sample)   Lower Body/Torso

Copy this sheet and file it with your fitness documents		Date: 8/1	Date: 8/2	Date: 8/3	Date: 8/4	Date: 8/5	Date: 8/6	Date: 8/7
Exercise: wall quarter squats page 71	RESIST:	Self	Self	Self				
	1st set	12	14	16				
	2nd set	12	14	16				
	3rd set	12	14	16				
Exercise: wall half squats page 71	RESIST:				Self	Self	Self	Self
	1st set				12	14	16	16
	2nd set				12	14	16	16
	3rd set				12	14	16	16
Exercise: leg abductions page 92	RESIST:	Self	Self	Self	Self	Self	Self	Self
	1st set	12 per leg	14 per leg	16 per leg	16 per leg	16 per leg	16 per leg	16 per leg
	2nd set	12 per leg	14 per leg	16 per leg	16 per leg	16 per leg	16 per leg	16 per leg
	3rd set	12 per leg	14 per leg	16 per leg	16 per leg	16 per leg	16 per leg	16 per leg
Exercise: heel raises page 91	RESIST:			Self	Self	Self	Self	Self
	1st set			12	14	16	16	16
	2nd set			12	14	16	16	16
	3rd set			12	14	16	16	16
Exercise: sitting leg raises page 83	RESIST:	Self	Self	Self				
	1st set	12 per leg	14 per leg	16 per leg				
	2nd set	12 per leg	14 per leg	16 per leg				
	3rd set	12 per leg	14 per leg	16 per leg				
Exercise: abs: sitting knee raises page 81	RESIST:	Self	Self	Self				
	1st set	12 per leg	14 per leg	16 per leg				
	2nd set	12 per leg	14 per leg	16 per leg				
	3rd set	12 per leg	14 per leg	16 per leg				
Exercise: simult. sitting knee raises page 72	RESIST:				Self	Self	Self	Self
	1st set				12	12	12	14
	2nd set				12	12	12	14
	3rd set				12	12	12	14

Program #1 (Sample) Upper Body/Torso

Copy this sheet and file it with your fitness documents		Date: 8/1	Date: 8/2	Date: 8/3	Date: 8/4	Date: 8/5	Date: 8/6	Date: 8/7
Exercise: wall push-ups page 72	RESIST:	Self	Self	Self	Self	Self	Self	Self
	1st set	8	12	14	16	16	16	16
	2nd set	8	10	12	14	16	16	16
	3rd set	8	10	12	14	16	16	16
Exercise: biceps curls page 104	RESIST*:	5 lbs	5 lbs	5 lbs	5 lbs	8 lbs	8 lbs	8 lbs
	1st set	8	10	12	12	8	10	12
	2nd set	8	10	12	12	8	10	12
	3rd set	8	10	12	12	8	10	12
Exercise: lateral arm raises page 103	RESIST:			Self	Self	Self	1.5 lbs	1.5 lbs
	1st set			8	10	12	8	10
	2nd set			8	10	12	8	10
	3rd set			8	10	12	8	10
Exercise: sitting arm abductions page 82	RESIST:	Self	Self	Self				
	1st set	8	10	12				
	2nd set	8	10	12				
	3rd set	8	10	12				
Exercise: one-arm rowing page 100	RESIST*:			5 lbs.	5 lbs.	5 lbs.	8 lbs.	8 lbs.
	1st set			8 per arm	10 per arm	12 per arm	8 per arm	10 per arm
	2nd set			8 per arm	10 per arm	12 per arm	8 per arm	10 per arm
	3rd set			8 per arm	10 per arm	12 per arm	8 per arm	10 per arm
Exercise: abs: sitting knee raises page 81	RESIST:	Self	Self	Self				
	1st set	12 per leg	14 per leg	16 per leg				
	2nd set	12 per leg	14 per leg	16 per leg				
	3rd set	12 per leg	14 per leg	16 per leg				
Exercise: simult. sitting knee raises page 72	RESIST:				Self	Self	Self	Self
	1st set				12	14	16	16
	2nd set				12	14	16	16
	3rd set				12	14	16	16

* Some seniors (especially women) may be more comfortable starting with 3-lb. weights and working up to 5-lb. weights.

Program #2: Somewhat Active Plus No Medical Problems

Let's assume you have no medical problems and that your doctor has cleared you for strength training. You are active and walk daily for about forty-five minutes. You garden from spring to late fall and spend winters in the south, where besides your daily walk you swim and occasionally play golf. Your lifestyle habits are good except for problems related to managing stress, but you have recognized the symptoms, identified the sources, and are well on your way to developing coping skills. Your chronological age is eighty, but your biological age—thanks to your regular physical activity, good nutrition, and steadily improving ability to cope with stress—is in the mid-seventies. You have noticed some loss of muscle and decrease in strength and want to embark on a strength-training program.

You went to your local YMCA for a fitness assessment. Your strength is average for your age, but your posture needs improvement. You have a tendency to hunch your back and to let your shoulders fall forward. The initial goal of your strength-training program should be to strengthen the muscles that keep your spine in a correct, neutral position and to stop your shoulders from hunching. To accomplish these things, the fitness professional doing the assessment recommended that you work on your middle trapeziuses, rhomboids, scapular stabilizers, and spinal erectors. The safest and most effective way to strengthen these muscles is to exercise with a stability ball on a daily basis.

Do the following three stability-ball exercises every day:

1. Lifting opposite arm and leg (page 86). Do eight to twelve repetitions in three sets. Between sets, rest on the ball with hands and feet on the floor, and gently rock back and forth for a couple of minutes as you remain relaxed.
2. Walk out (page 87). Repeat the exercise six to eight times in three sets. Between sets, gently rock back and forth on the ball, remaining relaxed.
3. Curl back (page 86). Do three sets of eight to twelve repetitions. Between sets, relax on the ball, gently rocking back and forth.

After a few weeks, increase the challenge of your stability-ball workout by increasing the number of repetitions in each set to fourteen or sixteen.

In addition to your stability-ball routine, each week you can do one session of lower-body/torso exercises and one session of upper-body/torso exercises. Do them on nonconsecutive days. See the sample charts that follow for ideas about how to structure these routines. Because you are fairly fit, the duration of each session can be thirty to forty-five minutes at the beginning. In a few months increase it to sixty minutes by adding additional exercises to both your lower-body/torso and upper-body/torso routines.

Program #2 (Sample) Stability-Ball Exercises

Copy this sheet and file it with your fitness documents		Date: 9/15	Date: 9/16	Date: 9/17	Date: 9/18	Date: 9/19	Date: 9/20	Date: 9/21
Exercise:	RESIST:	Self	Self	Self	Self	Self	Self	Self
lifting opposite arms and leg page 86	1st set	8	10	12	14	16	16	16
	2nd set	8	10	12	14	16	16	16
	3rd set	8	10	12	14	16	16	16
Exercise:	RESIST:	Self	Self	Self	Self	Self	Self	Self
walk out page 87	1st set	6	8	10	12	14	16	16
	2nd set	6	8	10	12	14	16	16
	3rd set	6	8	10	12	14	16	16
Exercise:	RESIST:	Self	Self	Self	Self	Self	Self	Self
extension or curl back page 86	1st set	8	10	12	14	16	16	16
	2nd set	8	10	12	14	16	16	16
	3rd set	8	10	12	14	16	16	16
Exercise:	RESIST:							
	1st set							
	2nd set							
	3rd set							
Exercise:	RESIST:							
	1st set							
	2nd set							
	3rd set							
Exercise:	RESIST:							
	1st set							
	2nd set							
	3rd set							
Exercise:	RESIST:							
	1st set							
	2nd set							
	3rd set							

Program #2 (Sample) Lower Body/Torso

Copy this sheet and file it with your fitness documents		Date: 9/15	Date: 9/16	Date: 9/17	Date: 9/18	Date: 9/19	Date: 9/20	Date: 9/21
Exercise: dumbbell squats page 90	RESIST*:	10 lbs	10 lbs	10 lbs	12 lbs	12 lbs	12 lbs	15 lbs
	1st set	8	10	12	8	10	12	8
	2nd set	8	10	12	8	10	12	8
	3rd set	8	10	12	8	10	12	8
Exercise: leg abduction page 92	RESIST:	Self	Self	Self	Self	Self	Self	Self
	1st set	8 per leg	10 per leg	12 per leg	14 per leg	16 per leg	16 per leg	16 per leg
	2nd set	8 per leg	10 per leg	12 per leg	14 per leg	16 per leg	16 per leg	16 per leg
	3rd set	8 per leg	10 per leg	12 per leg	14 per leg	16 per leg	16 per leg	16 per leg
Exercise: forward lunges page 93	RESIST:	Self	Self	Self	Self	Self	Self	Self
	1st set	8 per leg	10 per leg	12 per leg	14 per leg	16 per leg	16 per leg	16 per leg
	2nd set	8 per leg	10 per leg	12 per leg	14 per leg	16 per leg	16 per leg	16 per leg
	3rd set	8 per leg	10 per leg	12 per leg	14 per leg	16 per leg	16 per leg	16 per leg
Exercise: heel raises page 91	RESIST:	Self	Self	Self	Self	Self	Self	Self
	1st set	8	10	12	14	16	16	16
	2nd set	8	10	12	14	16	16	16
	3rd set	8	10	12	14	16	16	16
Exercise: leg adductions (stability ball) page 94	RESIST:	Ball	Ball	Ball	Ball	Ball	Ball	Ball
	1st set	8	10	12	14	16	16	16
	2nd set	8	10	12	14	16	16	16
	3rd set	8	10	12	14	16	16	16
Exercise: abs: trunk curls page 95	RESIST:	Self	Self	Self	Self	Self	Self	Self
	1st set	8	10	12	14	16	16	16
	2nd set	8	10	12	14	16	16	16
	3rd set	8	10	12	14	16	16	16
Exercise:	RESIST:							
	1st set							
	2nd set							
	3rd set							

* Some seniors (especially women) may be more comfortable starting with 3-lb. weights and working up to 5-lb. weights.

Program #2 (Sample)   Upper Body/Torso

Copy this sheet and file it with your fitness documents		Date: 9/15	Date: 9/16	Date: 9/17	Date: 9/18	Date: 9/19	Date: 9/20	Date: 9/21
Exercise:	RESIST*:	12 lbs	12 lbs	12 lbs	12 lbs	15 lbs	15 lbs	15 lbs
dumbbell chest press page 99	1st set	8	10	12	12	8	10	12
	2nd set	8	10	12	12	8	10	12
	3rd set	8	10	12	12	8	10	12
Exercise:	RESIST:	12 lbs	12 lbs	12 lbs	12 lbs	15 lbs	15 lbs	15 lbs
one-arm rowing page 100	1st set	8 per arm	10 per arm	12 per arm	12 per arm	8 per arm	10 per arm	12 per arm
	2nd set	8 per arm	10 per arm	12 per arm	12 per arm	8 per arm	10 per arm	12 per arm
	3rd set	8 per arm	10 per arm	12 per arm	12 per arm	8 per arm	10 per arm	12 per arm
Exercise:	RESIST:	10 lbs	10 lbs	10 lbs	12 lbs	12 lbs	12 lbs	12 lbs
dumbell biceps curls page 104	1st set	8	10	12	12	8	10	12
	2nd set	8	10	12	12	8	10	12
	3rd set	8	10	12	12	8	10	12
Exercise:	RESIST:	15 lbs	15 lbs	15 lbs	15 lbs	20 lbs	20 lbs	20 lbs
chest pullover page 102	1st set	8	10	12	12	8	10	12
	2nd set	8	10	12	12	8	10	12
	3rd set	8	10	12	12	8	10	12
Exercise:	RESIST:	8 lbs	8 lbs	8 lbs	8 lbs	10 lbs	10 lbs	10 lbs
dumbell lateral raise page 103	1st set	8	10	12	12	8	10	12
	2nd set	8	10	12	12	8	10	12
	3rd set	8	10	12	12	8	10	12
Exercise:	RESIST:	Self	Self	Self	Self	Self	Self	Self
abs: trunk curls page 95	1st set	10	12	14	16	16	16	16
	2nd set	10	12	14	16	16	16	16
	3rd set	10	12	14	16	16	16	16
Exercise:	RESIST:	Self	Self	Self	Self	Self	Self	Self
trunk cross curl with knee pull page 96	1st set	6	8	10	12	14	16	16
	2nd set	6	8	10	12	14	16	16
	3rd set	6	8	10	12	14	16	16

* Some seniors (especially women) may be more comfortable starting with 3-lb. weights and working up to 5-lb. weights.

9 | Beginning Exercises and Stability-Ball Exercises

Beginning Exercises

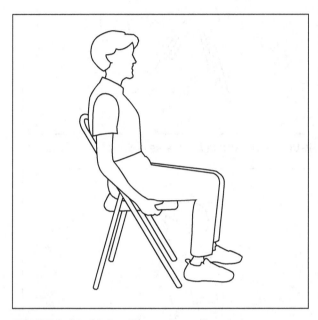

FIGURE 9.1A. *Sitting knee raise — Start*

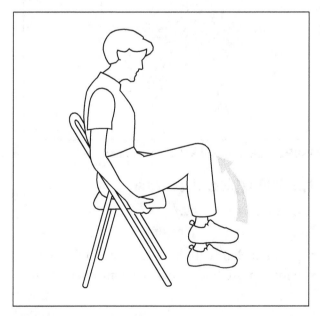

FIGURE 9.1B. *Sitting knee raise — Finish*

1. Sitting Knee Raise

Muscles participating:
Iliopsoas, abdominals

- Sit on a chair.
- Raise one bent knee toward your chest.
- Then lower the knee.
- Repeat with the other knee.

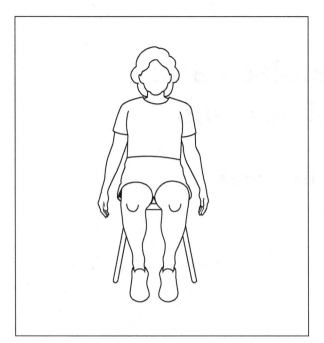

FIGURE 9.2A. *Sitting arm abduction — Start*

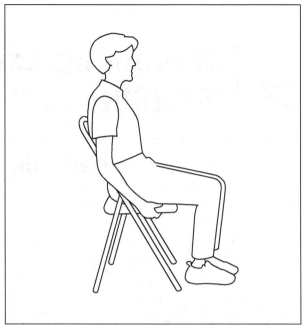

FIGURE 9.3A. *Sitting heel raise — Start*

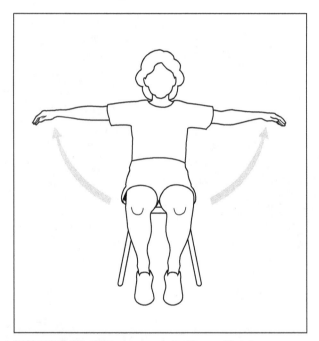

FIGURE 9.2B. *Sitting arm abduction — Finish*

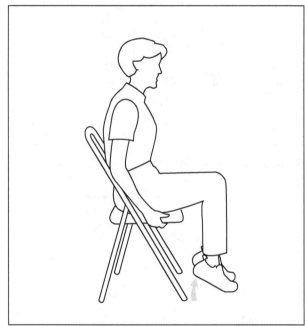

FIGURE 9.3B. *Sitting heel raise — Finish*

2. Sitting Arm Abduction

Muscles participating:
Deltoids, upper trapeziuses

- Sit on a chair with your arms hanging by your sides.
- Raise arms to the horizontal position.

3. Sitting Heel Raise

Muscles participating:
Calves (gastrocnemius, soleus)

- Sit on a chair with both feet flat on the floor.
- Slowly raise both heels in a controlled manner.

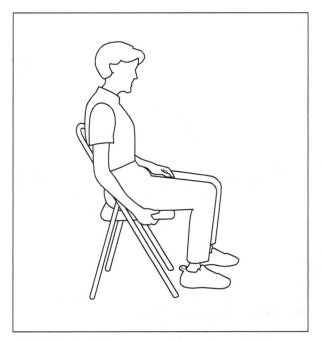

FIGURE 9.4A. *Sitting arm and leg raise — Start*

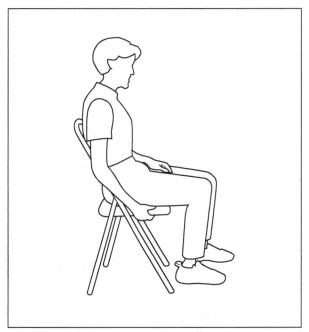

FIGURE 9.5A. *Sitting leg raise — Start*

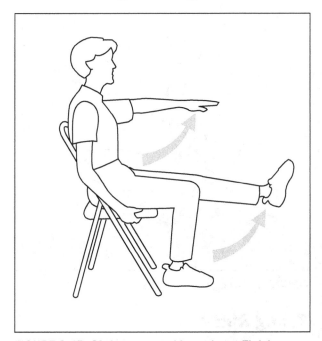

FIGURE 9.4B. *Sitting arm and leg raise — Finish*

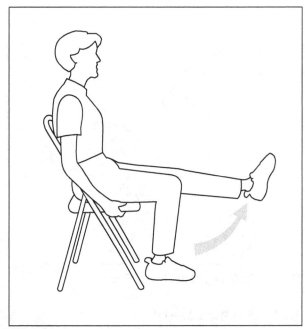

FIGURE 9.5B. *Sitting leg raise — Finish*

4. Sitting Arm and Leg Raise

Muscles participating:
Deltoids, quadriceps, iliopsoas

- Sit on a chair.
- Raise arm and leg on one side simultaneously.
- Lower the arm and leg.
- Repeat with the other side.

5. Sitting Leg Raise

Muscles participating:
Quadriceps, iliopsoas

- Sit on a chair.
- Slowly raise one leg in a controlled motion, extending it fully as you raise it.
- Lower it slowly.
- Repeat with the other leg.

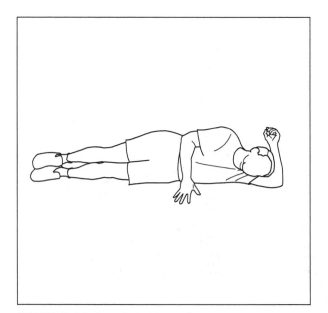

FIGURE 9.6A. *Leg abduction — Start*

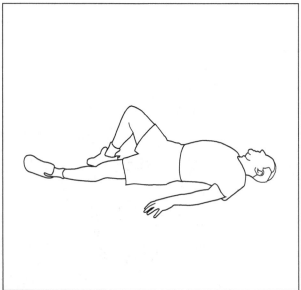

FIGURE 9.7A. *Leg raise — Start*

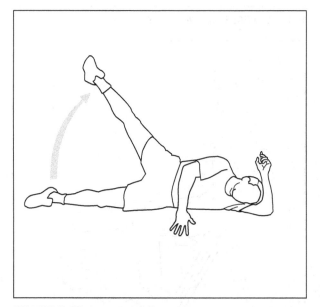

FIGURE 9.6B. *Leg abduction — Finish*

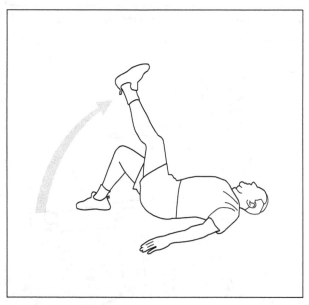

FIGURE 9.7B. *Leg raise — Finish*

6. Leg Abduction

Muscles participating:
Gluteus medius and minimus

- Lie on your side with one leg over the other and one arm under your head. Your other arm is flexed, with the hand flat on the floor.
- Slowly raise the top leg in a controlled motion as high as you can.
- Hold for a moment.
- Lower the leg slowly.

7. Leg Raise

Muscles participating:
Iliopsoas, quadriceps, abdominals

- Lie on the floor on your back with one leg extended and the other leg bent, foot flat on the floor.
- Slowly raise the extended leg in a controlled motion.
- Lower the leg.

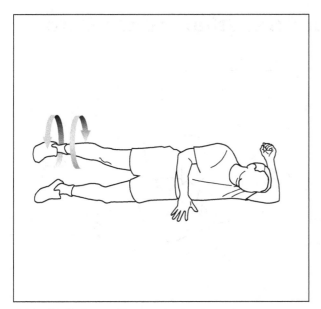

FIGURE 9.8. *Drawing circles with the leg*

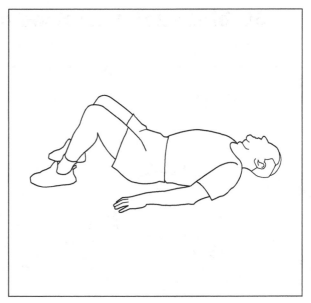

FIGURE 9.9A. *Pelvic tilt — Start*

8. Drawing Circles with the Leg

Muscles participating:
Gluteus medius and minimus

- Lie on your side with one arm under your head. Your other arm is flexed, with the hand flat on the floor.
- Lift the top leg and use it to "draw" circles in the air, first clockwise then counterclockwise. (One circle equals one repetition.)
- Repeat with the other leg.

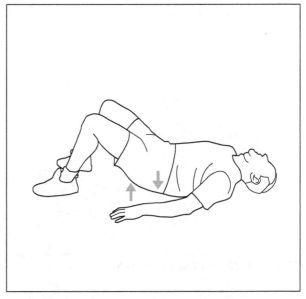

FIGURE 9.9B. *Pelvic tilt — Finish*

9. Pelvic Tilt

Muscles participating:
Abdominals, iliopsoas

- Lie on your back with your knees bent and your feet flat on the floor.
- Press the small of your back into the floor, contract the abdominals, and tilt the pelvis upward.
- Lower the pelvis and relax the abdominals.

Stability-Ball Exercises for Strengthening the Core

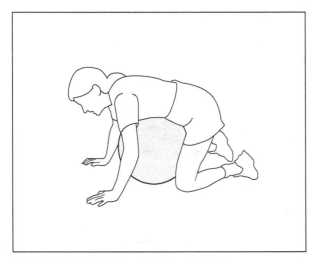

FIGURE 9.10A. *Curl back — Start*

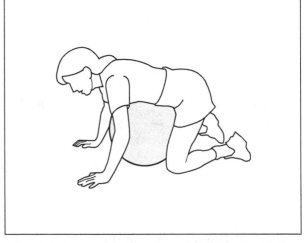

FIGURE 9.11A. *Lifting opposite arm and leg — Start*

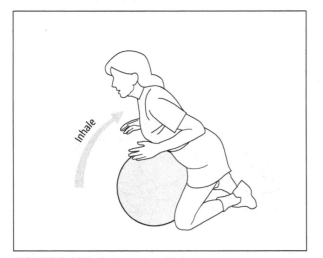

FIGURE 9.10B. *Curl back — Finish*

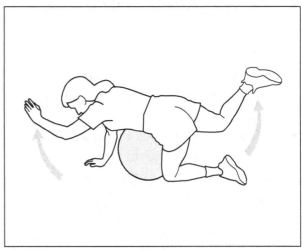

FIGURE 9.11B. *Lifting opposite arm and leg — Finish*

1. Curl Back

Muscles participating:
Quadratus lumborum spinal erectors, rhomboids, middle trapeziuses

- Crouch over the ball and position it between your knees.
- Press your pelvis into the ball and slowly raise your elbows above your back. Inhale during this movement.
- Maintain this position for a moment, then slowly return to the starting position as you exhale.

2. Lifting Opposite Arm and Leg

Muscles participating:
Scapular stabilizers, rotator cuff, hip extensors

- Position yourself over the ball and exhale.
- Press your abdomen and pelvis into the ball.
- Slowly and simultaneously raise one arm and the opposite leg while inhaling.
- Hold for a moment, lower, and exhale.
  - Repeat with the other arm and leg.

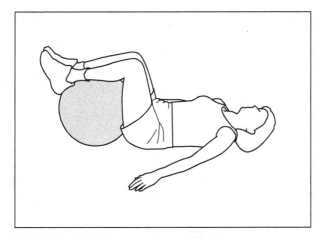

FIGURE 9.12A. *Hip extension — Start*

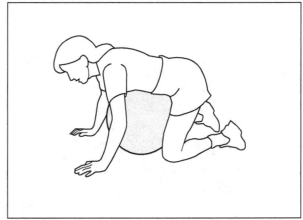

FIGURE 9.13A. *Walk out — Start*

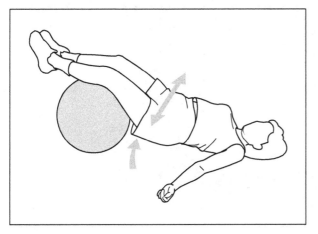

FIGURE 9.12B. *Hip extension — Finish*

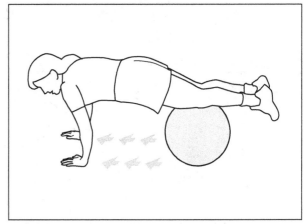

FIGURE 9.13B. *Walk out — Finish*

3. Hip Extension

Muscles participating:
Gluteals, quadratus lumborum, spinal erectors

- Lie on your back with legs resting on the ball.
- Inhale.
- Extend your hip by pressing your legs down on the ball and raising your buttocks off the floor.
- Exhale.
- When the hip is extended and the buttocks raised, move your hip slowly to the right and then to the left. Breathe regularly.
- Repeat this sideways motion four to six times.
- Lower your buttocks.

4. Walk Out

Muscles participating:
Rotator cuff, scapular stabilizers, triceps, abdominals

- Position yourself over the ball, with knees behind the ball.
- Using your arms, slowly propel yourself forward in small "walking steps," with the ball under your trunk and your legs raised.
- Slowly propel ("walk") yourself backward.

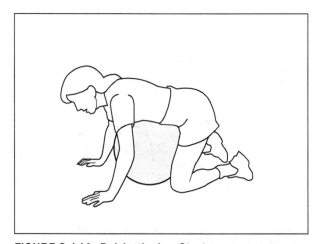

FIGURE 9.14A. *Pelvic clock — Start*

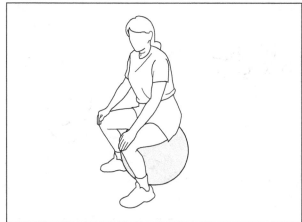

FIGURE 9.15A. *Pelvic circles — Start*

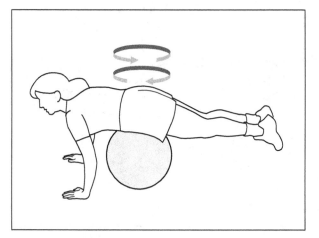

FIGURE 9.14B. *Pelvic clock — Finish*

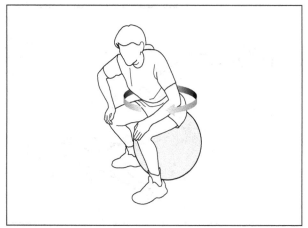

FIGURE 9.15B. *Pelvic circles — Finish*

5. Pelvic Clock

Muscles participating:
Scapular stabilizers, rotator cuff, deltoids, triceps, abdominals, pectorals, quadratus lumborum

- Position yourself on the ball with your knees behind the ball.
- Your hands should be flat on the floor, slightly farther apart than shoulder width. Using your arms, slowly propel ("walk") yourself forward until the ball is under your pelvis. Your legs are raised.
- "Draw" small clockwise circles with your pelvis on the ball; then "draw" counterclockwise circles. Use your arms and shoulders to assist with this movement.
- Slowly "walk" yourself backward.

6. Pelvic Circles

Muscles participating:
Abdominals, quadratus lumborum, spinal erectors

- Sit on the ball with your feet flat on the floor, wider than shoulder width apart.
- Rotate your pelvis clockwise a few times, then counterclockwise.

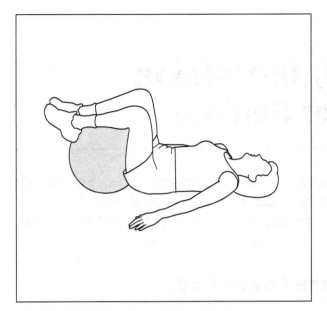

FIGURE 9.16A. *Bent-knee twist — Start*

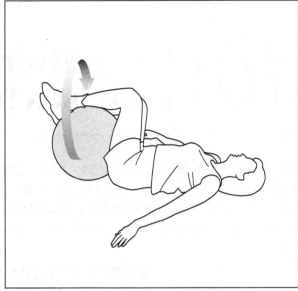

FIGURE 9.16C. *Bent-knee twist — Twist to the right*

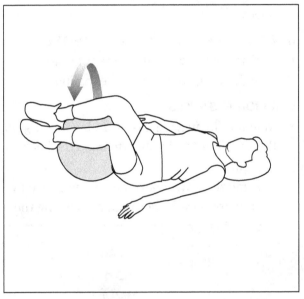

FIGURE 9.16B. *Bent-knee twist — Twist to the left*

7. Bent-Knee Twist

Muscles participating:

Anterior and posterior obliques, hamstrings

- Place legs on the ball and gently squeeze the ball against your butt.
- Squeeze the ball hard and twist your trunk to the left while lowering your knees to the left.
- Bring the ball back to the original position.
- Relax the squeeze.

- Repeat by twisting your trunk to the right while lowering your knees to the right.
- Bring the ball back to the original position.
- Relax the squeeze.

10 | Basic Strength-Training Exercises for Seniors

In this chapter I describe, step-by-step, how to perform some basic strength-training exercises. You can include them in your initial program according to your individual needs and abilities. If you start strength training after an extended period of sedentary life, choose only a few, less-difficult exercises. Add more and increase the level of difficulty gradually, as your strength improves.

Exercises for the Lower Body

1. Dumbbell Squat

Muscles participating:
Gluteals and quadriceps (prime movers); hamstrings, calves, spinal erectors, upper trapeziuses (secondary movers and postural stabilizers)

PREPARATIONS:
- Hold dumbbells so that your palms are facing your thighs.
- Position your feet so that they are parallel and shoulder width apart.
- Look straight ahead and adjust your posture so that your back is erect, your shoulders are back, and your weight is distributed evenly on both feet.
- Exhale fully.

DOWNWARD (NEGATIVE) MOVEMENT PHASE:
- Slowly lower into a squat as you inhale. Maintain correct posture while keeping your legs parallel. Squat only as far as you feel comfortable with. You can stop at any point. Never descend lower than the point where your derriere is level with your knees.

UPWARD (POSITIVE) MOVEMENT PHASE:
- Perform the upward movement by slowly straightening your legs and exhaling.

COMMON MISTAKES:
- Maintaining incorrect posture by drawing up the shoulders and failing to keep the back straight
- Starting the downward movement phase by leaning forward rather than by pushing the

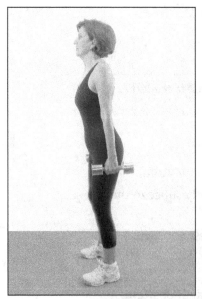

FIGURE 10.1A. *Dumbbell squat — Start*

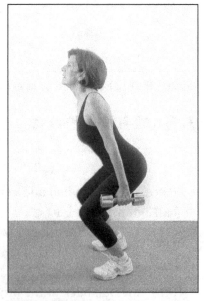

FIGURE 10.1B. *Dumbbell squat — Finish*

derriere back and bending the knees

- Pushing the knees inward or outward so that they are out of parallel position
- Raising the heels

EASIER VERSIONS:

- Perform the movement without resistance (without dumbbells), with hands on hips

and elbows drawn back.

- Stand up from a chair or bench with hands on hips and elbows drawn back.
- Stand with your feet about a foot away from a wall but with your derriere and elbows against the wall; slide them along the wall when you squat.

2. Heel Raises

Muscles participating:

Calves (prime movers); quadriceps, hamstrings (assisting)

PREPARATIONS:

- Stand in front of a wall; place your palms on the wall at shoulder height and shoulder width apart.
- Step back and fully extend your arms until you are leaning against the wall at a slight angle.

- Look straight ahead, raise your chest, draw in your abdomen, then inhale.

UPWARD (POSITIVE) MOVEMENT PHASE:

- Start exhaling and slowly raise your heels until you are on the balls of your feet. Hold the position for a moment.

DOWNWARD (NEGATIVE) MOVEMENT PHASE:

- Slowly lower your heels as you inhale. (If you slightly bend your knees, there will be more muscle action from the soleus than from the gastrocnemius muscle.)

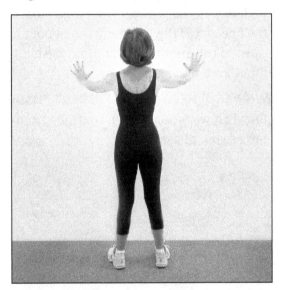

FIGURE 10.2A. *Heel raises — Start*

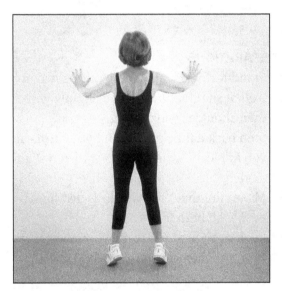

FIGURE 10.2C. *Heel raises — Finish*

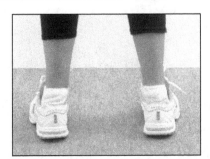

FIGURE 10.2B. *Heel raises — Start (close-up)*

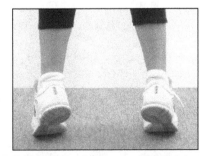

FIGURE 10.2D. *Heel raises — Finish (close-up)*

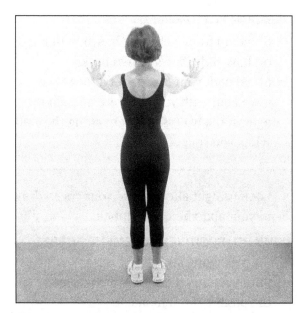

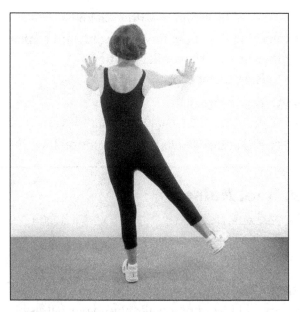

FIGURE 10.3A. *Leg abduction (lateral leg raise) — Start*

FIGURE 10.3B. *Leg abduction (lateral leg raise) — Finish*

3. Leg Abduction (Lateral Leg Raise)

Muscles participating:
Gluteus medius and minimus

PREPARATIONS:

- Stand facing a wall; place your palms on the wall at shoulder height and slightly wider than shoulder width apart.
- Step back a little and extend your arms until you are leaning against the wall at a slight angle.
- Make sure that your weight is distributed evenly on both feet.
- Look straight ahead, raise your chest, draw in your abdomen, then inhale.

UPWARD (POSITIVE) MOVEMENT PHASE:

- Raise one straightened leg laterally (to the side) as you exhale. Raise it slowly and as high as you can without straining. Make sure the knee faces the wall rather than pointing upward toward the ceiling. Hold the leg lifted for a moment.

DOWNWARD (NEGATIVE) MOVEMENT PHASE:

- Slowly lower your leg in a controlled manner as you inhale.

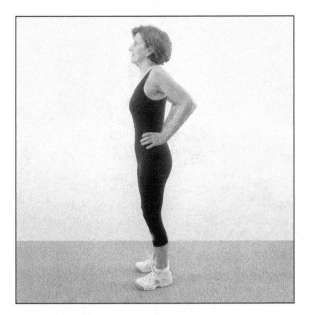

FIGURE 10.4A. *Forward lunge — Start*

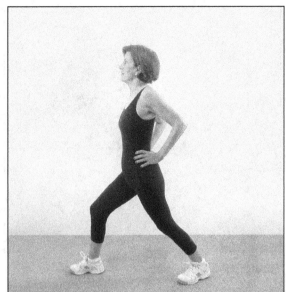

FIGURE 10.4B. *Forward lunge — Finish*

4. Forward Lunge

Muscles participating:
Quadriceps and gluteals (primary movers);
hamstrings and calves (secondary movers)

PREPARATIONS:

- Stand erect and look straight ahead with shoulders back and chest up. Your arms hang freely at your sides with palms facing your thighs. Option: hands on hips.

FORWARD (NEGATIVE) MOVEMENT PHASE:

- Lift one leg and lunge forward as you inhale. Make sure that you stay within your comfortable range of motion. Land on the full sur- face of your foot. At the end of the forward lunge, your knee should be above the toes of your foot. Pause for a moment.

BACKWARD (POSITIVE) MOVEMENT PHASE:

- Push back and exhale, bringing your feet to- gether.

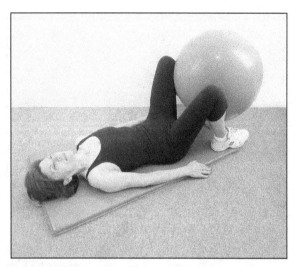

FIGURE 10.5A. *Leg adduction — Start*

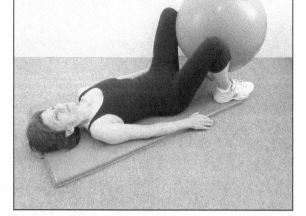

FIGURE 10.5B. *Leg adduction — Finish*

5. Leg Adduction

Muscles participating:
Adductor magnus, adductor brevis, adductor longus, and gracilis

PREPARATIONS:

- Lie on an exercise mat with your knees flexed at 90°. Your feet should be flat on the floor somewhat wider than shoulder width apart. Place the exercise ball between your knees.

INWARD (POSITIVE) MOVEMENT PHASE:

- Inhale. Start exhaling as you press the small of your back down into the exercise mat while slowly squeezing the exercise ball with your knees in a controlled manner. Hold the squeeze for a moment at the end of the motion.

OUTWARD (NEGATIVE) MOVEMENT PHASE:

- Slowly release your knees' pressure on the ball as you inhale.

Exercises for the Trunk

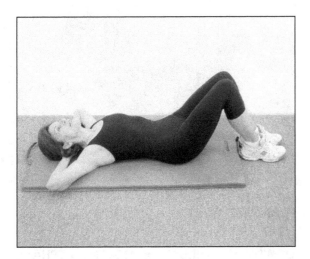

FIGURE 10.6A. *Trunk curls — Start*

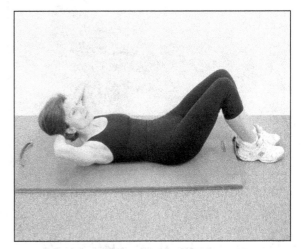

FIGURE 10.6B. *Trunk curls — Finish*

1. Trunk Curls

Muscles participating: **Rectus abdominus**

PREPARATIONS:

- Lie on your back on a mat with your knees flexed at 110°–120°. Put your hands under the nape of your neck to maintain the neutral alignment of your neck. Inhale.

UPWARD (POSITIVE) MOVEMENT PHASE:

- Press the small of your back into the mat while contracting your abs and slowly raising your shoulders. Hold for a moment. Exhale as you perform this upward movement.

DOWNWARD (NEGATIVE MOVEMENT) PHASE:

- Slowly lower your shoulders as you inhale.

CAUTION:

- Avoid using your hands to raise your neck. Trying to gain momentum by raising your neck with your hands will result in incorrect and less effective execution of the exercise and may also harm your neck.

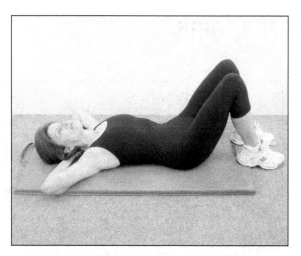

FIGURE 10.7A. *Trunk cross curl with knee pull — Start*

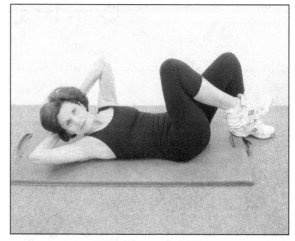

FIGURE 10.7B. *Trunk cross curl with knee pull — Finish*

2. Trunk Cross Curl with Knee Pull

Muscles participating:
Abdominal obliques, rectus abdominus

PREPARATIONS:

• Lie on your back on a mat with your knees bent at 110°–120°. Put your hands under the nape of your neck to support the neutral alignment of your neck. Inhale.

UPWARD (POSITIVE) MOVEMENT PHASE:

• Press the small of your back slowly into the mat while raising your left knee and right shoulder simultaneously. Rotate your trunk slowly so that your right elbow moves toward your left knee and, if you can, touch your left knee with your right elbow. Hold for a moment. Exhale during this upward movement. (After the downward movement, repeat the motion with your right knee and left shoulder, moving your left elbow toward your right knee.)

DOWNWARD (NEGATIVE) MOVEMENT PHASE:

• Slowly and simultaneously lower your left knee and your right elbow back to the starting position. Inhale during the downward phase.

CAUTION:

• Avoid using your arms to assist in rotating your trunk upwards. Your hands behind your neck should do no more than support the neutral alignment of your neck. Gaining any momentum by raising your neck with your hands will result in incorrect execution of the exercise and may also strain your neck.

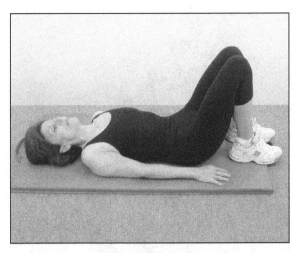

FIGURE 10.8A. *Assisted bent-knee trunk curl —
Start*

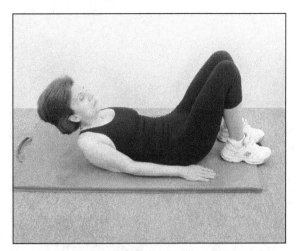

FIGURE 10.8B. *Assisted bent-knee trunk curl —
Finish*

3. Assisted Bent-Knee Trunk Curl

Muscles participating:
Rectus abdominus

PREPARATIONS:
- Lie on your back on a mat with your knees
  bent at 110°–120°. Your arms should be on
  the floor at your sides with the palms facing
  down. Inhale.

UPWARD (POSITIVE) MOVEMENT PHASE:
- Press the small of your back into the mat and
  contract your abs while pushing your elbows
  and forearms downward against the mat and
  slowly curling your trunk upward in a controlled manner. Exhale during this upward
  movement. Pause for a moment at the top of
  the motion.

DOWNWARD (NEGATIVE) MOVEMENT PHASE:
- Slowly lower your trunk back onto the mat
  in a controlled manner. Inhale during this
  downward movement.

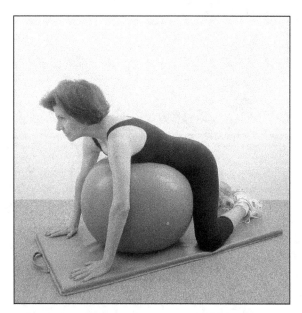

FIGURE 10.9A. *Back extension (stability ball) — Start*

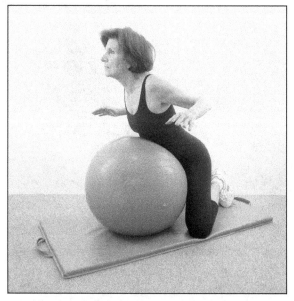

FIGURE 10.9B. *Back extension (stability ball) — Finish*

4. Back Extension (Stability Ball)

Muscles participating:

Spinal erectors, quadratus lumborum, middle trapeziuses

PREPARATIONS:

- Place a stability ball under your trunk so that your chest, abdomen, and pelvis are fully supported by the ball. Hug the ball with your knees and arms. Your hands rest on the floor.

UPWARD (POSITIVE) MOVEMENT PHASE:

- Press your pelvis and abdomen against the ball while slowly raising your elbows above your back as you arch your back, slowly extending it. Inhale during the upward movement. Hold this position with elbows drawn back and shoulder blades contracted.

DOWNWARD (NEGATIVE) MOVEMENT PHASE:

- Slowly lower your trunk onto the ball in a controlled manner. Exhale during this downward movement.

CAUTION:

- This exercise must be done in a controlled and coordinated manner. Bouncing up or down on the ball will only compromise the effectiveness of the exercise and may strain your body as well.

Exercises for the Upper Body

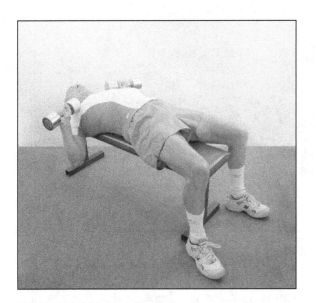

FIGURE 10.10A. *Dumbbell chest press — Start*

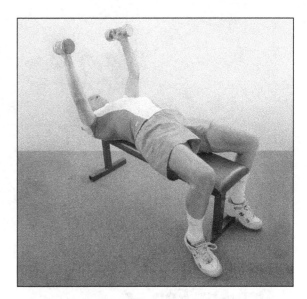

FIGURE 10.10B. *Dumbbell chest press — Finish*

1. Dumbbell Chest Press

Muscles participating:
Pectoralis major, anterior deltoids, triceps

PREPARATIONS:
- Select two dumbbells of equal weight. Sit on one end of a flat bench so that your feet are shoulder width apart on the floor. Hold the dumbbells so that they are resting on your upper thighs.
- Slowly lower your back onto the bench while raising the weights up to your chest so that they almost touch your chest. Your palms should face upward.
- In this position your legs are straddling the bench, your knees are bent at 90°, and your feet are flat on the floor. Inhale.

UPWARD (POSITIVE) MOVEMENT PHASE:
- Raise both dumbbells in a slow and controlled manner until your arms are fully extended. Exhale during the upward movement. Make sure that you keep your head, shoulders, and buttocks in contact with the bench. Hold for a moment.

DOWNWARD (NEGATIVE) MOVEMENT PHASE:
- Slowly lower both dumbbells until they touch the sides of your chest. Inhale during this downward movement.

CAUTION:
- Do not let your head hang off the bench.
- Do not arch your back when you raise the dumbbells.
- Do not bounce the dumbbells against your chest when you lower them and then use the momentum to raise them.
- If you feel any pain in your lower back (lumbar area), avoid straining it by resting your feet on a stool in front of the bench. If you feel any pain in the shoulder area, stop the downward movement slightly before the chest.

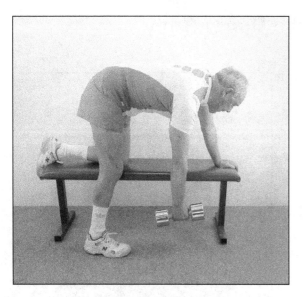

FIGURE 10.11A. *One-arm rowing — Start*

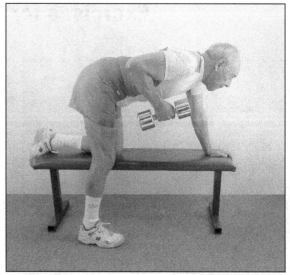

FIGURE 10.11B. *One-arm rowing — Finish*

2. One-Arm Rowing

Muscles participating:
Latissimus dorsi, biceps

PREPARATIONS:

- Place a dumbbell on the floor along one side of the bench and stand behind the dumbbell. Place the knee that is closest to the bench on the bench. Keep the other leg straight and your foot flat on the floor. Lean forward and grip the end of the bench with one hand. With your other hand, reach down for the dumbbell and hold it so that your back is straight and flat and your arms are fully extended.

UPWARD (POSITIVE) MOVEMENT PHASE:

- Slowly raise the dumbbell toward your hip in a controlled manner. Hold the position at the end of the movement for a moment.

DOWNWARD (NEGATIVE) MOVEMENT PHASE:

- Slowly lower the dumbbell to the starting position.

BREATHING:

- One-arm rowing is one of the exercises in which the (positive) effort is toward the center of the body. During these sorts of exercises, many prefer to inhale through the upward movement because it makes the chest a more solid platform for the exercise. You may want to experiment with inhaling through the positive (upward) movement and exhaling during the negative (downward) movement. If you find this confusing, then stick with the general rule of exhaling during the positive (upward) movement.

CAUTION:

- Do not hunch or overextend your back.
- Place your knee on the bench directly under your hip and keep the leg you stand on parallel with it to ensure that your back is not strained.
- Do not overextend the downward movement.

3. Dumbbell Chest Fly

Muscles participating:
Pectoralis major, anterior deltoid, biceps

PREPARATIONS:

- Select two dumbbells of equal weight. Sit on one end of a flat bench so that your feet are shoulder width apart on the floor. Hold the

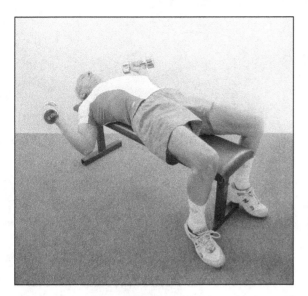

FIGURE 10.12A. *Dumbbell chest fly — Start*

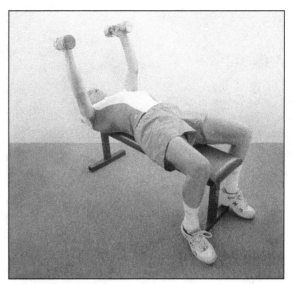

FIGURE 10.12B. *Dumbbell chest fly — Finish*

dumbbells so that they rest on your upper thighs.

- Slowly lower your back onto the bench while raising the weights to your chest. Hold them about twelve inches away from the sides of your shoulders at shoulder level with your palms facing each other. Your elbows should be bent a little less than 90°.

- In this position your legs are straddling the bench, your knees are bent at 90°, and your feet are flat on the floor. Your head, shoulders, and buttocks should be in contact with the bench. Do not overextend your back.

- Inhale.

UPWARD (POSITIVE) MOVEMENT PHASE:

- Slowly raise the two dumbbells in a controlled manner until the dumbbells touch each other. Your elbows should stay slightly bent at the top of the movement.

- Exhale during the upward movement. Hold for a moment.

DOWNWARD (NEGATIVE) MOVEMENT PHASE:

- Slowly pull the dumbbells away from each other in a slow and controlled manner and lower them while decreasing the angle at which your elbows are bent until they are bent a little less then 90° at the end of the motion, that is, when the dumbbells are level with the top of your chest.

- Inhale during the downward movement.

CAUTION:

- Do not let your head hang off the bench.

- Do not arch back when you raise the dumbbells.

- Make sure that your elbows are slightly bent at the top of the movement and bent to about 90° at the bottom. It is very important that your elbows never exceed 90° at the bottom of the movement. If you extend (straighten) your elbows to more than 90°, you may strain your shoulders.

- Always keep your wrists straight. Make sure that your hands are always in line with your forearms. It is a common mistake to put strain on the sensitive wrist joints by bending them.

- Never lower the dumbbells below the level of your chest, and never raise them suddenly with a countermovement.

- If you feel strain in the chest or shoulder area, decrease the movement range so that the dumbbells are above the level of your chest at the bottom of the motion.

- If you feel pain in the lower back, rest your feet on a stool in front of the bench.

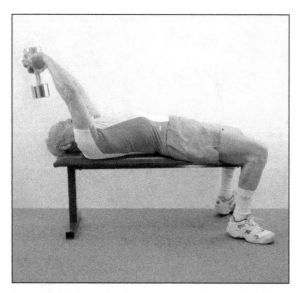

FIGURE 10.13A. *Chest pullover — Start*

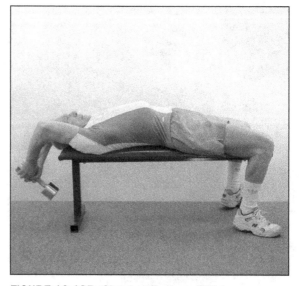

FIGURE 10.13B. *Chest pullover — Finish*

4. Chest Pullover

Muscles participating:
Latissimus dorsi, triceps

PREPARATIONS:
- Select one dumbbell. Sit on the end of a bench with both hands holding the shaft of the dumbbell parallel with your torso, palms facing each other.
- Slowly lower yourself onto your back and raise the dumbbell above your chest.
- Put both thumbs under the shaft and cup both hands, one over the other, around one end of the dumbbell. Slowly lift the dumbbell with both hands and hold it with arms slightly flexed directly above your head.
- Your head is positioned at the end of the bench, your back and buttocks are flat on the bench, your feet are flat on the floor, and your knees are bent at 90°.

DOWNWARD (NEGATIVE) MOVEMENT PHASE:
- With elbows kept parallel, slowly lower the dumbbell behind your head. Make sure that your back is not overextended.
- Inhale during the downward movement. Hold for a moment.

UPWARD (POSITIVE) MOVEMENT PHASE:
- Press your lower back into the bench slightly while slowly lifting the dumbbell above your head. While lifting, keep extending your elbows until they are just slightly bent at the top of the motion, that is, directly above your head. Keep your elbows parallel.
- Exhale during the upward movement.

CAUTION:
- Always keep your elbows parallel; do not push them outward. Gradually decrease the angle of the elbows so that you start with slightly flexed elbows and finish with elbows bent at 90° at the end of the motion behind your head.
- Lowering the dumbbell with elbows pushed outward or with straightened elbows will strain your shoulders.
- Make sure (as with every exercise) that you do not bounce back with a sudden counter-movement. Rather, bring the dumbbell to a halt at the bottom of the movement, hold it for a moment, then slowly return it to the starting position.
- Do not let your head hang off the bench.
- It is a common mistake to arch the back while doing the chest pullover. This can strain your back. If you feel any pain in your back, put a stool under your feet.

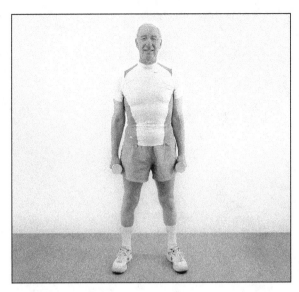

FIGURE 10.14A. *Dumbbell lateral raise — Start*

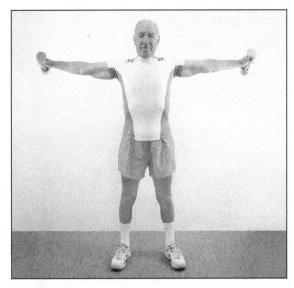

FIGURE 10.14B. *Dumbbell lateral raise — Finish*

5. Dumbbell Lateral Raise

Muscles participating:
Deltoids, upper trapeziuses

PREPARATIONS:

- Select a pair of dumbbells. Stand with your feet shoulder width apart and knees slightly flexed. Hold the dumbbells with arms slightly flexed so that your palms are facing your thighs.
- Make sure that your chest and chin are up. Do not push your head forward, hunch your back, or let your shoulders fall forward.

UPWARD (POSITIVE) MOVEMENT PHASE:

- Slowly raise your arms sideways until the dumbbells are level with your shoulders and your arms are parallel with the floor. During the upward movement, keep your elbows slightly flexed.
- During this upward movement, keep your chest and chin up, and your shoulders and head aligned with your body rather than slumped forward. Do not hunch as you lift the dumbbells.
- Your wrists must also be kept in neutral position; that is, they should be aligned with your forearms rather than bent.
- Exhale during the upward movement.

DOWNWARD (NEGATIVE) MOVEMENT PHASE:

- Slowly lower the dumbbells in a controlled manner to the starting position.
- Inhale during the downward movement.

CAUTION:

- Never attempt to lift the dumbbells above shoulder level. If you feel pain in the shoulders, you should stop the upward movement before the dumbbells are level with the shoulders.
- Do not allow your shoulders to lift during the upward movement. Keep the shoulder blades drawn down and back throughout the exercise.
- It is also a common mistake to let the dumbbells hang with your wrists bent. The hands should always be aligned with the forearms, without a bend at the wrist in any direction.

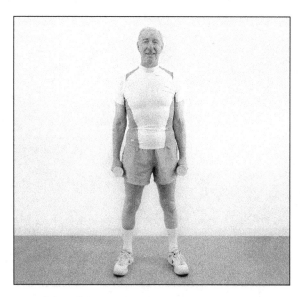

FIGURE 10.15A. *Dumbbell biceps curl — Start*

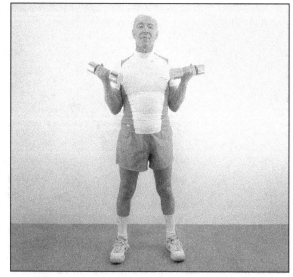

FIGURE 10.15B. *Dumbbell biceps curl — Finish*

6. Dumbbell Biceps Curl

Muscles participating:
biceps, brachialis, radiobrachialis

PREPARATIONS:
- Select a pair of dumbbells and hold them with your arms at your sides and the palms facing the thighs.
- Stand with your feet hip width apart and your knees slightly bent. Stand erect, with your chest and chin up and your shoulders level.

UPWARD (POSITIVE) MOVEMENT PHASE:
- Slowly raise the dumbbells, rotating your wrists upward and keeping the elbows close to your sides and the upper arms aligned with your chest. When the dumbbells are at shoulder level, your palms are facing your shoulders.

DOWNWARD (NEGATIVE) MOVEMENT PHASE:
- Slowly lower the dumbbells simultaneously in a controlled manner.

BREATHING:
- The biceps curl is another exercise in which the positive movement is performed in the direction of the body. Inhaling while raising the dumbbells expands the chest, which will provide a more solid platform for the exercise. You can try inhaling during either the positive (upward) or the negative (downward) movement phase and see which pattern feels better. If this is confusing, stick to exhaling during the positive movement phase and inhaling during the negative movement phase.

CAUTION:
- Keep your back straight throughout the exercise. Do not lean backward or forward.
- Pause at the bottom of the motion for a moment; do not swing the dumbbells like a pendulum.
- Keep the elbows close to your sides and the upper arms aligned with the chest. Do not raise your elbows as you perform the upward movement.
- Wrists should always be aligned with the forearms in a neutral position; they should not be bent.

Basic Stretches

The function of stretches is to elongate and relax the muscles and connective tissues, and to increase range of motion at the joints. In this section I describe some basic stretches that are safe and can be learned with relative ease. They can be applied after each exercise and/or after the completion of each exercise session.

1. Achilles Stretch

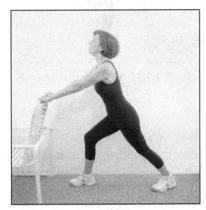

FIGURE 10.16. *Achilles stretch*

PURPOSE:

- The Achilles stretch elongates the Achilles tendon and the calf muscles. Do the Achilles stretch after heel raises, squats, and lunges. You should also do it after a long walk.

EXECUTING THE STRETCH:

- Place your hands against something stable, like a wall, a table, or the back of a chair.
- Slowly move your left leg forward, bend it, and move your right leg back, keeping it fully extended. Bend the front leg further and keep both heels firmly on the ground.
- Hold the stretch for about ten seconds. Feel the stretch in the Achilles tendon and in the calves.
- Switch legs and repeat.

2. Piriformis Stretch

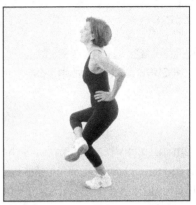

FIGURE 10.17. *Piriformis stretch*

PURPOSE:

- The piriformis stretch elongates the piriformis and gluteus medius muscles. It also improves hip-joint mobility. You should do this stretch after leg abductions and squats.

EXECUTING THE STRETCH:

- Stand next to a wall and support yourself by placing your right hand on the wall and leaning slightly against it.
- Bend your left (supporting) leg. Place your right leg—which should be bent at about 90°—in such a way so that the bottom portion of your right leg rests just above the knee of your left leg. The ankle of the right leg should be slightly outside of the thigh of the left leg.
- Slowly lower your body by bending the left leg even more. Feel the stretch at the right side of your hip, buttock, and thigh. To increase the stretch, push your buttock back slowly.
- Hold the stretch for about ten seconds.
- Repeat the same stretch by reversing the position of your legs.

3. Hamstrings Stretch

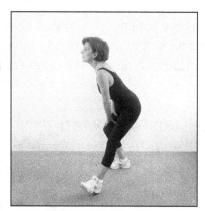

FIGURE 10.18. *Hamstrings stretch*

PURPOSE:

- The hamstrings stretch elongates the hamstring muscles, located along the back of the leg. It should be performed after squats and lunges and after a long walk.

EXECUTING THE STRETCH:

- Step forward with your left leg and bend your right leg. With both hands above the knee of the right leg, bend forward a little.
- Fully extend your left leg and curl your toes back (dorsiflexion) so that only your heel touches the ground. Keep your back straight, press your left heel into the ground, and push your buttocks back. Feel the stretch in the back of your left leg; hold it for about ten seconds.
- Repeat the stretch with legs reversed.

4. Quadriceps Stretch

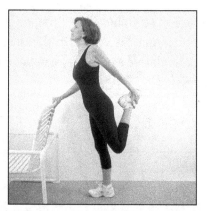

FIGURE 10.19. *Quadriceps stretch*

PURPOSE:

- Elongates the quadriceps and iliopsoas (groin) muscles and improves hip mobility. Perform this stretch after squats and lunges and after a long walk.

EXECUTING THE STRETCH:

- Support yourself by leaning against a wall, a table, or the back of a chair. Lift your left foot by bending your knee, and hold onto your foot with your left hand. Slowly start pulling your foot up and moving your left knee behind the fully extended right leg.
- Feel the stretch in the front of your left leg and in the groin. Hold the stretch for about ten seconds.
- Reverse legs and repeat.

5. Triceps Stretch

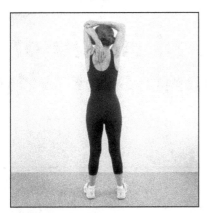

FIGURE 10.20. *Triceps stretch*

PURPOSE:

- Elongates the triceps muscles, which run between the elbow and the shoulder in the back of the arm. Do the stretch after the chest press and push-ups, and after any other exercises that involve the extension (straightening) of the arms against resistance.

EXECUTING THE STRETCH:

- Lift your left arm above your head, bend it, and lower your hand until the palm of your hand touches the top of your back. Lift your right arm and wrap your right hand around the elbow of the left arm.
- Slowly pull the elbow in the direction of the center of your body. Feel the stretch between the elbow and the shoulder of the left arm. Hold it for about ten seconds.
- Reverse your arms and repeat.

6. Pectoralis/Biceps Stretch

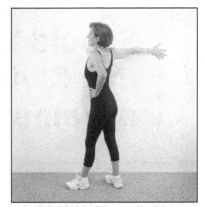

FIGURE 10.21. *Pectoralis/biceps stretch*

PURPOSE:

- Elongates the chest, anterior deltoid, and biceps muscles, and improves range of motion at shoulder joint. Do this stretch after chest flies, biceps curls, and push-ups.

EXECUTING THE STRETCH:

- Stand with your right side parallel to a wall, and your right foot about six inches from the wall. Step forward with your left leg and draw your right arm up behind your back until it is at shoulder height. Your right arm should be fully extended and the palm of your hand should be pressed against the wall.
- Slowly rotate your trunk to the left. Feel the stretch in the right chest muscles, right shoulder, and biceps. Hold for about ten seconds.
- Reverse positions and repeat.

• • • • •

You can learn more advanced stretches as you progress with your strength-training program. But if you perform these basic stretches on a regular basis after each exercise session, you will keep your muscles relaxed and will also experience a gradual improvement in your range of motion.

11 | Should You Train at Home or in a Club? By Yourself or with a Trainer?

In this chapter we will carefully weigh the pros and cons of training at home or in a fitness club, as well as the pros and cons of hiring a personal trainer or exercising on your own. These are very important practical decisions that may influence the way you begin and continue with your strength-training program. It is worthwhile to invest some time and effort in considering these choices because they can affect both the process and the outcome.

Home Training vs. Training at a Fitness Club

If you live in a condo or apartment complex with exercise facilities, or in a home with enough room to provide space for exercising, you may want to choose home training. Although at home you will probably lack the wide range and variety of exercise equipment that is available in fitness clubs, you may enjoy the convenience of not having to travel, park, change clothes, exercise, shower, change back into your regular clothes, and return home. On average, unless the fitness club is within easy walking distance, one spends more time on travel than on exercise.

I train most of my clients in their homes. Even though the exercise area is often small and the equipment sometimes consists only of the basics, they get just as much out of each session as the clients I train in the best-equipped fitness clubs. Some of my home clients let me set up their training facility and hire me to design a program and demonstrate the exercises, and then they continue strength training on their own. When I visit them periodically to teach new exercises and plan further progression, they seem satisfied with working out at home. If you feel more comfortable at home and want the convenience of not having to join and travel to a fitness club, home training is certainly a viable choice.

On the other hand, if you are more comfortable in a fitness club and think you will take advantage of the wide range and variety of exercise equipment and entertainment, and if you enjoy the company of other members and want to try the various services (massage, fitness seminars) and classes (from yoga to Pilates) offered at most clubs, then joining a fitness club is a sensible choice.

Before signing a membership agreement, you must make sure that you know everything you need to about the club, for example:

- Is the location convenient?
- How accessible is parking?
- What are the hours of operation?
- Take a tour during the time of the day when you will likely attend the club to see if the atmosphere is pleasant, too crowded, or too noisy (with music blasting from speakers, etc.).
- Check for cleanliness and orderliness in the exercise areas, locker rooms, and restrooms.
- Are the employees and members are polite, considerate, and courteous?
- Check the availability, variety, condition, and layout of training equipment.
- Ask about the rules of conduct.
- Ask about the qualifications of fitness personnel.

You can ask for a one-month complimentary membership to allow you to try out the club's facilities before deciding whether to join. If a one-month complimentary membership is unavailable, ask for a few free passes, or just sign up for a month. Take advantage of this introductory period to ask other members if they are happy with the services they receive.

If you decide to join, take the membership agreement home, read the small print, and ask questions. If you are dissatisfied with the clarity of any of the answers you receive, don't hesitate to investigate further. Clubs usually charge an initiation fee, want automatic bank withdrawals, and impose various other contractual commitments. You should sign up only if you are completely satisfied with the terms.

Equipment in a Fitness Club

Most fitness clubs have a wide variety of strength-training equipment. The range and complexity of machines available in a club may overwhelm someone who is unfamiliar with them. As a club member, you are entitled to a demonstration of various fitness machines by qualified personnel. Take advantage of this opportunity; ask for an initial demo of the basic machines. Make notes as you watch and listen, and do not hesitate to ask questions.

Start simply. It is better to become well acquainted with a few basic, easy-to-use machines for the legs, trunk, and upper body than to have a superficial knowledge of too many machines. A few weeks later you may want to extend your knowledge. Ask for another demo of the more complicated pieces of equipment. Always be sure to learn how to adjust the machines for a perfect fit and how to load and unload them safely. Before you begin working with the machines in any fitness club, review the section in Chapter 7 titled "Preparations for a Safe Training Environment" to refresh your memory about how to avoid accidents that can lead to injury.

Exercising on Your Own vs. Exercising with a Personal Trainer

Although most seniors are better off working with a personal trainer or fitness professional when they embark on a strength-training program, training on your own may be a viable choice. If you cannot afford the services of a trainer on an ongoing basis, you can always start by purchasing a few sessions. This way, at least your initial program can be custom-designed for you by a professional. Make good use of those first few sessions; learn how to execute the exercises safely and effectively. If you cannot afford the expense of even a few sessions with a personal trainer, you can buy strength-training books and videos, take advantage of the services of various community centers, or learn from friends who are already exercising. This method could result in slower progress, and you may have to cope with the mistakes that accompany learning to exercise by trial and error.

If, on the other hand, hiring a personal trainer in a club or at home is an option for you, there are certain important steps you should take before doing so. Personal training is still largely an unregulated profession. There are trainers with excellent qualifications from internationally recognized institutions with very high standards, such as the National Strength and Conditioning Association (NSCA) and the American Council on Exercise (ACE). In these institutions, the education, theoretical knowledge, and practical knowledge of candidates is thoroughly tested before they are granted certification and become qualified to train others. To meet the strict recertification processes that both organizations periodically require of their members, trainers must dedicate a lot of effort to keeping their knowledge current and relevant through continuing education.

There are a few trainers out there who obtained their certification via mail order from self-declared "institutions" or who took a short course provided by a local community center and became "certified" by passing a low-level exam. It is very important to make sure that the personal trainer you intend to hire is certified by either the NSCA or ACE or by an accredited college. Unqualified trainers may fail to help you achieve your goals and may even cause you harm.

Both the NSCA and ACE provide referral services for personal trainers in specific geographical areas. Here is contact info:

- NSCA—*website:* www.nsca-lift.org; *phone:* (800) 815-6826 or (719) 632-6722
- ACE—*website:* www.acefitness.org; *phone:* (800) 825-3636 or (858) 279-8227

After making certain that the prospective personal trainer is well qualified and certified by ACE or NSCA, or has a diploma from an accredited college, I would highly recommend that you do some further checking to make sure that he or she has the necessary experience and disposition to train mature adults. You want qualities such as thoughtfulness, attentiveness, carefulness, dedication, and loyalty to clients, as well as compatibility. These are qualities beyond the ability of any organization that certifies personal trainers to measure. When you interview prospective trainers, it is important to ask for and to check referrals. You should also ask about their experience in working with seniors. You may want to know what professional publications they read. These can range from bulletins issued by ACE and NSCA to the *Journal of Aging and Physical Activity* or *Physician and Sports Medicine.* Working with a more knowledgeable trainer improves the odds of your obtaining better results.

During the interview, you should pay attention to how thoroughly the prospective trainer asks you about your medical history and condition, medications you may be taking, and your fitness history and status. Does the trainer want your doctor's clearance and a fitness assessment? Ask for an initial program so you can determine whether the targets of that program are realistic and reasonable. Watch out for unrealistic promises— they are always a sign of carelessness.

I highly recommend that before making any long-term commitment, you ask your prospective trainer for either a paid or a complimentary session in order to decide if he or she demonstrates sufficient care and patience in teaching you how to perform the various exercises safely, correctly, and effectively, with attention to proper breathing and posture. Also pay attention to whether the trainer checks to make sure that the equipment and the immediate surroundings are safe so that your session will take place without injury caused by a careless accident.

Find out if the trainer has the personality and attitude necessary for motivating and encouraging you and helping you through periods of stagnation, inertia, and the occasional decline in your commitment to exercising. See if the trainer

- is focused and disciplined and is also able to inspire focus and discipline in you
- has a positive attitude that will motivate you to achieve your goals
- has the energy, vitality, and inner drive to give the training process momentum, direction, and focus
- can recognize certain negative and positive factors in you and has the skills to influence and interact so that the positive factors prevail
- can provide the necessary emotional support to keep you focused on achieving your goals

When I teach trainers, I find that most of them have the necessary knowledge to be good personal trainers, but only a few have the positive attitude and energy needed to inspire and motivate their clients. Few have effective psychological and interpersonal skills. However hard it is to find such a trainer, the effort invested in searching for one will be paid back handsomely. Never resign yourself to a situation in which you are paying a trainer just to have someone to attend your sessions. Keep asking around, and sooner or later you will find a trainer who will be your guide and partner on your journey to a stronger and fitter body.

12 | Real-Life Examples to Teach and Inspire

In this chapter I use real stories from some of my clients to illustrate how to commence and progress with a comprehensive and personalized strength-training program. The stories can serve as inspiration and education. They can also help you to be prepared for some of the problems—from mental blocks to injuries—people sometimes encounter when following a regular training regimen. All of the people profiled in this chapter are seniors ranging in age from fifty-five to eighty-five.

Harriet

When Harriet retired she wished to live her life to the fullest. She came to the realization that everything she wanted to do—from playing the piano to traveling, gardening, and playing tennis—required a strong fitness base. She was healthy, with no restrictions or contraindications to exercising. At the same time, her state of fitness was below her potential.

Harriet's physical assets were good flexibility, good coordination, and a well-proportioned body with healthy bones, joints, and muscles. Her liabilities were some postural problems, a certain degree of muscle asymmetry, and insufficient lean muscle mass, which resulted in inferior strength. Her psychological assets were an absolute commitment to playing by the rules in order to improve her fitness, a great sense of discipline, and the ability to patiently persist until things worked out. As an additional bonus, she was eager to learn about her body, about good eating habits, about training in general, and about strength training in particular. In short, she was ready to apply the same positive attitude and persistence to her physical training that had made her very successful in her professional career.

We agreed that the most important goal was to improve her posture and dynamic muscle balance through strength training. We began with three parallel programs. The first program was corrective; the exercises consisted mostly of stability-ball exercises to strengthen her postural stabilizers. That is, due to weak scapular (shoulder blade) stabilizers, her shoulders fell forward, and weak spinal erectors resulted in an incorrect curvature/alignment of the spine. We started with exercises designed to improve these specific problems with her posture. Once the stronger core muscles began improving her posture, she progressed to a wider range of stability-ball exercises that, besides correcting her posture, improved the overall strength of her trunk as well as her functional skills such as balance and coordination.

The method we adopted with this exercise modality was to start with three or four essential exercises that she did under supervision until she perfected them. Then she continued doing those exercises on her own, and during our sessions we learned and added new ones to her routine until she had two comprehensive stability-ball training routines consisting of twelve exercises each, which she did on alternating days.

Harriet's second program, which accompanied the stability-ball training, was a daily walk at a brisk pace for about thirty to forty-five minutes. It was not just simple fast walking; she also paid attention to correct posture, efficient gait, and proper breathing.

In tandem with the corrective program aimed at improving posture and muscle balance and the aerobic program to improve cardiovascular fitness, we also started on a progressive strength-training program. Three times a week, we exercised with free weights to improve her general strength. We were very cautious with the pace of progression. The emphasis was on improving quality, form, and technical correctness rather than on increasing the frequency, duration, and intensity of the workouts. Exercises had to be performed with proper posture, breathing, and coordination, and in their full range of motion.

We applied the following method to maintain progression:

- For each of the exercises that made up her initial strength-training program, we determined the ideal resistance. To be on the safe side, we chose a resistance against which she was able to perform each exercise eight times, both with technical correctness and without straining. In order to give her body plenty of opportunity to learn and imprint the correct execution of each exercise, we had her perform three consecutive sets, with stretching between each set.

- As I have mentioned, the focus was on perfecting Harriet's technique. The exercises had to be performed slowly and in a controlled manner, with fluid and coordinated movements, and in their full range of motion. We also made sure that she maintained both correct posture and breathing pattern throughout each exercise.

- Once all aspects of technique were perfected, we gradually increased the number of repetitions from eight to ten to twelve to fourteen, and finally to sixteen for each set.
- Once Harriet could easily and correctly perform three sets of sixteen repetitions of each exercise in this initial program, instead of following the usual method of increasing resistance by 5 percent, we learned new exercises. We did not want to fall into the trap of strengthening only certain muscle groups while neglecting others.
- Once we had increased the variety and complexity of strength-training exercises to a degree where every important muscle group in Harriet's body received regular and systematic training, then we increased resistance by 5 percent (and at the same time reduced the number of repetitions to eight per set).

Because Harriet wanted to excel in tennis, we made sure that her trunk muscles were strong. It is in the trunk where various forces find the platform from which to initiate motion, and to enhance or cancel out each other. That is, the trunk must be strong because it must provide a solid platform for the various forces initiating different movements. It is very important that the muscles of the trunk be able not only to generate force, but also to withstand the torque and the shearing forces of the sudden countermovements common in tennis. We added more exercises to improve the strength of the muscles in her midsection. We also progressed to performing complex structural exercises, which improve muscle strength in the context of function (rather than in isolation).

Harriet maintained her interest in continuing to learn about training, nutrition, and stress management. Thanks to her commitment, discipline, focus, and determination to improve her fitness, after four years of training she managed to reduce her biological age by more than ten years. Her tennis improved to such a degree that she is able to compete against younger players. Her improved strength and posture positively affected her piano playing. Now she does most of her training on her own and remains as committed and disciplined as ever.

I found that Harriet's greatest strength was her absolute and unwavering commitment to improving her fitness.

James

James was about fifty pounds overweight and very out of shape. Due to a combination of bad eating habits, inactivity, and excess weight, he had high blood pressure and a narrowing of the coronary arteries. Before starting any serious training, James had to reduce his weight. Even his ability to walk for any extended period of time at a pace that could have been considered aerobic was compromised by the extra pounds he carried. His breathing was shallow, frequent, irregular, and inefficient because of the large deposit of subcutaneous fat in his stomach area.

Once James' initial assessments were completed, it was obvious that he had to do more than gradually improve his eating habits. We agreed that the number-one goal was reducing his weight. Until he consulted an excellent nutritionist, who refined the Spartan diet I immediately imposed on him, he ate fresh and steamed green vegetables and vegetable juices that were low in calories and very high in fiber. (To increase the fiber content of the vegetable juices, he added freshly ground flaxseed.) I told him to immediately eliminate the saturated fats and trans-fats that might entirely close his already badly narrowed coronary arteries. He also had to eliminate simple carbohydrates and every carbohydrate that was above thirty in the glycemic index, as well as processed foods and red meat. He was supposed to eat very small portions six or seven times a day.

I instructed James to walk daily without straining himself. The establishment of an efficient but relaxed breathing pattern was the most important aspect of his cardiovascular training. At the same time, we embarked on a comprehensive strength-training program. The idea was to combine a low-calorie, high-fiber diet; moderate aerobic exercise; and moderate strength training (which would build muscle, a metabolically very active tissue). Such a program would reduce his weight and blood pressure and progressively improve his capacity to train. We did strength training three times a week. He had a solid muscle base, but due to inactivity and overeating and the resulting obesity, his muscles were stiff and dysfunctional, able to produce only uncoordinated movements within a seriously restricted range of motion.

At the beginning, James experienced muscle soreness for weeks, even if we worked with relatively light weights. However, he persisted. His muscles responded well, and through a series of positive adaptations they became stronger and more functional. A few months later he started sea kayaking.

Due to the combination of dramatically improved eating habits, regular aerobic exercise, strength training (resulting in an active and functional musculature), and a new interest in a healthy and inspiring activity such as sea kayaking, James lost thirty pounds in six months. In a year his blood pressure was normal. Subsequent medical examinations showed a gradual improvement in the diameter of his coronary arteries. After several tests confirmed his increased ability to train, we added snowshoeing to his winter aerobic-exercise regimen. In his strength-training program, we focused on improving his muscle endurance by increasing the number of repetitions to twenty or more for each set.

James perfected his kayaking skills and improved his muscle endurance to such a degree that, after a year and a half of training, he was able to paddle at racing speed for 4.5 miles as a member of a masters quadrathlon team. He also went on several kayaking trips to the Northern Ontario lakes, where he was able to paddle for hours in rough water.

James' strength was his ability to recognize that his lifestyle habits were leading to a disaster and to take immediate action. His assets were his commitment to change, his persistence in continuing his exercise program, and his embracing of good lifestyle habits. He was ultimately able to achieve a lot more than he'd ever envisioned when he'd originally decided to lose a few pounds.

Mary and Norman

Mary and Norman are a wonderful couple. I worked with Mary first. She was frail, and, due to inactivity, her strength to function and perform movements was seriously compromised. Her inactivity resulted in low functional abilities, muscle atrophy, and osteoporosis. Her strengths were the ability to recognize that she had to make substantial and immediate changes in her sedentary lifestyle and a commitment to work patiently and consistently on her general goal of becoming more fit. She was eager to learn. She was very precise in documenting, recording, and monitoring her daily activities and her body's responses to training. This helped her to work out independently after a few initial sessions. We got together only periodically to assess her achievements, to widen the range of her exercise programs, and to plan further progression.

Initially, we designed and she learned a stability-ball program that helped her improve her core strength and coordinative skills safely and comprehensively. Once she perfected her daily routine, we embarked on a weight-training program of various antigravitational, weight-bearing exercises to improve bone mass and bone mineral density.

Mary enjoyed both the process of working toward her goals and achieving them. Her progress was gradual and steady. Slowly, her bones, joints, and muscles became noticeably stronger, and her functional abilities improved. Mary's dedication became an inspiration for her husband, Norman, who also began to exercise.

Norman was overweight and had high blood pressure, and his level of strength and aerobic fitness were far below his potential. His flexibility and posture were at a point where they seriously affected his ability to function.

Following his wife's example, he was just as persistent and consistent in his pursuit of improved fitness. In a year, not only did he lose weight, but his blood pressure became normal, and the dizziness and headaches he had experienced subsided. Whereas a few years ago he could not even imagine doing so, he now walks to his office daily and climbs stairs. Norman and Mary mutually encourage and motivate one another. They both reduced their biological age by at least ten years and enjoy the quality of life they deserve.

It is interesting to mention that with the few husband-and-wife couples I have trained, both the recognition that inactivity (and the resulting lack of physical fitness) was the single most important obstacle to maintaining their quality of life as well as the decision to do something about it originated with the wives. Husbands followed their wives' example after seeing the results.

Roberta

Roberta had serious rheumatoid arthritis and high blood pressure, and she was overweight. She had just recovered from cancer and from the deleterious effects of chemotherapy, extreme fatigue, overall weakness, and a compromised immune system. Her capacity to move and to function properly was severely restricted. Add to this her poor posture, ineffective gait, and restricted range of motion, and her prospects for a fit, healthy, active lifestyle were not encouraging. Roberta also led a very demanding, stressful, but physically inactive life. Her ability to cope with stress was almost nonexistent, and her attempts to manage stress were ineffective and counterproductive.

We started with a stability-ball program. Because of her high blood pressure, we avoided exercises such as the back extension that had to be performed in the prone position, which would have put pressure on her chest and abdomen. In concert with the stability exercises, we initiated a program of beginning strength-training exercises. Roberta worked out each day, alternating the stability-ball program and the beginning strength-training program. She also walked daily at a comfortable pace for twenty-five to thirty minutes. As her strength improved, we added increasingly complex exercises to her two programs. We also added various breathing exercises.

I explained to her that the effects of proper exercise are as much mental as they are physical—that when she exercises, she must focus on every aspect of correct form, breathing, and posture and shut out everything else. Focus is key. She should regard her entire program as a form of natural therapy.

Roberta's sense of discipline, perseverance, and keen attention to every detail of correct form paid off. Her improvements were spectacular. In less than six months her functional abilities, strength, range of motion, posture, and gait improved significantly. She lost fifteen pounds and reduced her biological age by five years.

Barb

Barb was overweight, her strength and aerobic capacity were far below her potential, and she had problems with joint flexibility. She realized that her fitness had to be improved when she decided to climb the highest mountain in the southern hemisphere. She knew that she lacked both the strength and the aerobic endurance to accomplish such a feat. She had only about three months to get herself into shape.

Barb had good potential that was unrealized because of her bad lifestyle habits; her terrible eating habits were the primary culprit in destroying her health and fitness. I recognized that her enthusiasm for the pursuit of her goal of climbing the mountain was a strong asset that would motivate her to accept a very strict and demanding nutritional and exercise regimen. To achieve her target, she could be persuaded to commit herself to playing by the rules. I had the impression that she had neither the discipline nor the patience to persist and stay on course without being inspired by a dramatic and immediate goal.

I told her that she had to follow precisely every prescription in her exercise and nutritional regimen because in order to perform the task ahead of her, her training had to push the limits of her body's ability to adapt. I told her that one step over the maximum amount of physical stress that her body was able to absorb and react to in a healthy manner would mean injury or burnout or both. This might not only put an end to her goal of climbing the mountain, but might also adversely affect her health.

We started immediately with strength training. We focused on antigravitational, weight-bearing exercises, such as squats, and we quickly progressed to cleans (a complex structural exercise) because she had to be able to lift and carry fifty pounds of climbing and camping equipment at high altitude. Her aerobic training consisted of fast walking on a treadmill. Instead of going for higher speed, we increased the angle of the treadmill as her strength and endurance improved.

Barb also had to change her eating habits, which were some of the worst I have ever seen; her meals consisted of all kinds of simple, processed carbohydrates, chocolate, and ice cream. It was late in the afternoon when we had our first meeting. My expression as I listened to the list of "foods" she had been abusing her body with must have betrayed my shock, because even before I had the opportunity to comment, she asked me when I wanted her to change her eating habits. I told her that "starting as of tomorrow" she had to change everything. I gave her a list specifying what she could eat and how much.

Her poor eating habits and total lack of discipline in resisting bad foods became the grounds for the first serious conflict among the many that followed. Because I told her that she had to change her eating habits "as of tomorrow," she took advantage of the twelve hours at her disposal to eat about three boxes of chocolates (the last of the Christmas candy) that were "lying around" her home.

To cut the story short, Barb did an excellent job with her climbing expedition, although her group failed to reach the summit because of bad weather. Her fitness and health improved dramatically. She took up kayaking, and within just three years her team of master athletes won two consecutive quadrathlon World Cup events, and she won several individual gold, silver, and bronze medals at Canadian and U.S. masters championships.

It was Barb's motivation, drive, competitive spirit, and enthusiasm that helped her achieve these incredible improvements in her quality of life. However, she still lacks the discipline, patience, and persistence needed to maintain and improve her health and fitness independently. Regardless, her example shows that even if you lack many of the qualities usually needed to achieve lasting favorable change, a reliance on one or two positive traits can overcome the disadvantages that stem from many unfavorable and counterproductive attitudes.

• • • • •

Use these case studies to inspire you on your journey toward a strong and health body, whatever your age and physical condition may be. See your doctor, take a fitness test, use the knowledge you've gained from reading this book, set your sights on a reasonable goal, and draw up an initial program that will lead you there. Do your first wall push-up and your first wall squat. Through increased strength, energy, and vitality, you will enjoy the rewards of your efforts in a few months.

13 | What Are You Waiting For?

The combination of inactivity, unhealthy eating habits, and the inability to cope with stress is the underlying cause of the physical decline that reduces our ability to enjoy life and to function independently as we get older. In fact, this mixture of unhealthy habits is notorious for reducing the quality of life of every age group in our society. On the other hand, everyone knows, intellectually or theoretically at least, the benefits of regular physical activity, healthy nutrition, and effective stress-management techniques.

Unfortunately, realizing the disadvantage or the advantage of something does not necessarily guarantee that constructive change or action will happen. Recognizing and comprehending is one thing; applying such knowledge in a practically useful manner is quite another. Between recognition and action lies a mental inertia that must be overcome.

I find that the inability to act *now*—which leads to endless postponements of the day when we commit ourselves to a cause—is the number-one reason for the lethargy and resignation that keep people from embarking on the journey that will lead to a better life. You have only one life to live. Why not make it the best and most enjoyable life you can?

What are some of the most common excuses I hear when I talk to older adults who are sedentary and overweight, but still unwilling to make that first decisive step? And what are my answers to those excuses?

"I'm Too Tired"

The less active you are, the longer you continue your bad eating habits, and the longer you delay dealing effectively with your stress, the more tired you will feel. The physical fatigue you feel is the result of inefficient circulation, stiff joints, and atrophied muscles. Your body is deprived of wholesome, quality nutrients. Stress takes away the energy you need to act.

Give lifestyle change a try. Take a walk and breathe. Do a few exercises. Eat healthy foods. If a doctor told you that taking a little white pill for thirty days would make you feel better, would you do it? Well, try exercise for thirty days. You will have more energy and will feel better. Once you have experienced a better lifestyle, you will be encouraged to continue and enjoy further gains.

"I Have No Time"

Examine the way you spend your days. Put your priorities in order. Eliminate the useless, the unproductive, and the nonsensical. You will be surprised at the amount of time freed up for training. The time you allot to exercise is your best investment. If you think that you cannot make time for exercise now, then be sure to make plenty of time for illnesses and hospitals later.

"I've Gotten to the Point Where I Am Unable to Effect a Change"

How do you know? You may be experiencing plateaus and burnouts because of an ill-designed program. Perhaps you are not performing the exercises with correct technique. You may be doing too little or too much.

If properly trained, everyone possesses the potential for improvement. If you fail to experience improvement and progression, see your doctor and consult a health-and-fitness professional. Let them show you how to effect change, how to draw on reserves that have never been properly utilized, how to find abilities where you see none. The last thing you ever should want to do is to resign yourself to the fact that something has not worked out and then to blame yourself for something that has nothing to do with your ability to succeed.

"I Tried, but I Didn't Have the Motivation to Go On"

If you don't succeed at first, keep persisting in a different manner. There are many roads that lead to fitness. Find your own.

Whatever road you choose, first commit yourself to making a change. Sign a self-contract. Specify and visualize your goals. Develop a plan to achieve them. Record and document the process—every step of it. Notice and appreciate your accomplishments, even the small ones. Remember that change occurs slowly, degree by degree.

Always think in terms of success instead of fearing failure. Every step you walk is a successful step, and every set of exercises you complete is a building block leading to a better and potentially magnificent edifice.

Constantly visualize yourself as healthy, fit, and strong. With your sights set on this goal, your heart and lungs will work better and your muscles will have extra strength to move you in that direction.

Listen to "can-do" motivational tapes and speeches. Learn how to encourage yourself with positive self-talk.

Seek out the company of like-minded people. Consider joining groups involved in recreational activities. Go to your local community center, YMCA/YWCA, or fitness club and see what they have to offer.

Reward yourself for persisting and achieving your targets. Go on a special trip. Buy that fancy mountain bike, the best walking shoes, the most comfortable and functional workout attire.

Don't wait for a moment. The more you postpone signing your self-contract and completing and recording your first set of exercises, the less likely you will be to begin after you put this book back on the bookshelf. Take that important first step now, and the second and third will follow naturally. Before you know it, you will be on your way to becoming the stronger and fitter person you have always wanted to be.

Worksheets

Behavior-Change Commitment Contract

I, _____, will begin my behavior-change program immediately and will incorporate the following into my daily routine:

1. I will pay attention to physical, behavioral, mental, and emotional signs of stress. I will become aware of and record my typical adverse reactions to stress, which may include everything from overeating to negative feelings.

2. I will begin to identify the *sources* of stress in my life and learn to be aware of them as they occur.

3. I will steadily work on improving my personal skills to cope with stress that results in fear, impulsiveness, anxiety, anger, preoccupation, and other negative feelings by

    a. working on building a positive mindset that includes changing perceptions, reactions, and being more reflective rather than reactive
    b. using breathing, relaxing, meditating, reading, listening to music, etc., to prevent and cope with stress
    c. constantly reviewing and appreciating the progress I am making and rewarding myself for making that progress
    d. enlisting the services of a professional counselor if I need outside support to do any of the above

4. I will work for change by taking small, manageable steps, rather than setting myself up for disappointment by trying to make sweeping changes.

_____   _____

SIGNATURE   DATE

Stress-Management Strategies

1. I listen to what my body is telling me. I learn to recognize the following signs of stress:

   - Muscle tightness
   - Slumped posture
   - Shaky hands
   - Sweating and/or night sweating
   - Headaches
   - Dry mouth
   - Rapid and shallow breathing
   - Lack of energy
   - Strained face

2. I am aware of the following behavioral signals of stress and their sources:

Signal	Identify Source
Talking to myself	_____
Arguing with people who aren't present	_____
Overeating/rushed eating	_____
Swearing	_____
Outbursts of anger	_____
Nagging others	_____
Increase in bad habits	_____
Withdrawing	_____
Working more and making mistakes	_____

3. I am aware of the following emotional signs of stress and their sources:

Signal	Identify Source
Fear	_____
Anger	_____
Worry	_____
Loss of sense of humor	_____
Irritation	_____

4. I employ the following strategies to manage my stress:

   a. Change my perception of things; acquire a sense of humor
   b. Reduce ambitions, lower expectations, become more realistic and accepting
   c. Learn to say no
   d. Get adequate sleep and rest
   e. Do deep breathing and use various relaxation techniques
   f. Seek counsel
   g. Others (write them here)

Behavioral Balance Sheet

Under the "Comments" columns, note when you feel each emotion (see the first example)

Positive	Comments	Negative	Comments
1. Sense of humor	e.g., I laugh at myself when I make a mistake.	1. Fear	e.g., I feel fear when I go for a checkup.
1. Sense of humor		1. Fear	
2. Calm		2. Anxiety	
3. Ability to reflect		3. Nervousness	
4. Ability to say no		4. Outrage	
5. Assertiveness		5. Indignation	
6. Optimism		6. Preoccupation	
7. Patience		7. Impatience	
8. Disipline		8. Pessimism	
9. Awareness		9. Annoyance	
10. Ability to let go		10. Worry	

Exercise/Lifestyle Commitment Contract

I, _____, pledge that

- I will do strength training three times a week on the following nonconsecutive days: _____, _____, and _____.

- I will adhere to the appropriate guidelines for strength training, including proper warm-up, correct execution of exercises, stretching, and cooldown.

- I will walk briskly at least thirty minutes daily to improve and maintain my cardiovascular fitness, and I will practice breathing exercises twice a day.

- In order to maximize my improvements and to fully realize my potential, I will systematically improve my lifestyle habits in the areas of nutrition and stress management, practice breathing exercises twice a day, and give myself opportunities to relax.

- My short-term goals for the next three months are the following:

  a. Lose _____ lbs.
  b. Be able to _____
  c. Be able to _____

- My long-term goals for the year are the following:

  a. Lose _____ lbs.
  b. Lower my blood pressure to _____
  c. Be able to _____
  d. Be able to _____
  e. Be able to _____

- I will keep a daily record of my activities.

- Every day I will reaffirm my commitment to doing all of the above.

- I will find ways of rewarding myself for every improvement.

_____   _____

SIGNATURE   DATE

Program # *Lower Body/Torso*

Copy this sheet and file it with your fitness documents		Date:	Date:	Date:	Date:	Date:	Date:	Date:
Exercise:	RESIST:							
	1st set							
	2nd set							
	3rd set							
Exercise:	RESIST:							
	1st set							
	2nd set							
	3rd set							
Exercise:	RESIST:							
	1st set							
	2nd set							
	3rd set							
Exercise:	RESIST:							
	1st set							
	2nd set							
	3rd set							
Exercise:	RESIST:							
	1st set							
	2nd set							
	3rd set							
Exercise:	RESIST:							
	1st set							
	2nd set							
	3rd set							
Exercise:	RESIST:							
	1st set							
	2nd set							
	3rd set							

Program # Upper Body/Torso

Copy this sheet and file it with your fitness documents		Date:	Date:	Date:	Date:	Date:	Date:	Date:
Exercise:	RESIST:							
	1st set							
	2nd set							
	3rd set							
Exercise:	RESIST:							
	1st set							
	2nd set							
	3rd set							
Exercise:	RESIST:							
	1st set							
	2nd set							
	3rd set							
Exercise:	RESIST:							
	1st set							
	2nd set							
	3rd set							
Exercise:	RESIST:							
	1st set							
	2nd set							
	3rd set							
Exercise:	RESIST:							
	1st set							
	2nd set							
	3rd set							
Exercise:	RESIST:							
	1st set							
	2nd set							
	3rd set							

Program #   Stability-Ball Exercises

Copy this sheet and file it with your fitness documents		Date:	Date:	Date:	Date:	Date:	Date:	Date:
Exercise:	RESIST:							
	1st set							
	2nd set							
	3rd set							
Exercise:	RESIST:							
	1st set							
	2nd set							
	3rd set							
Exercise:	RESIST:							
	1st set							
	2nd set							
	3rd set							
Exercise:	RESIST:							
	1st set							
	2nd set							
	3rd set							
Exercise:	RESIST:							
	1st set							
	2nd set							
	3rd set							
Exercise:	RESIST:							
	1st set							
	2nd set							
	3rd set							
Exercise:	RESIST:							
	1st set							
	2nd set							
	3rd set							

Recommended Reading

Allen, Lynn, editor. *Active Older Adults.* Champaign, IL: Human Kinetics, 1999.

Bouchard, Claude, et al., editors. *Exercise, Fitness and Health: A Consensus of Current Knowledge.* Champaign, IL: Human Kinetics, 1990.

Cotton, Richard T., editor. *Exercise for Older Adults.* San Diego, CA: American Council on Exercise, 1998.

Shephard, Roy J. *Aging, Physical Activity and Health.* Champaign, IL: Human Kinetics, 1997.

Index

Entries in italics refer to exercises described in the text.

CPSIA information can be obtained
at www.ICGtesting.com
Printed in the USA
JSHW041026240920
8179JS00005B/219

9 780897 934787